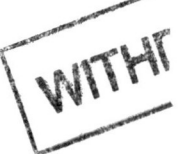

To all the husbands, lovers, partners and friends who have supported women through troubled hormonal times

Contents

PART ONE

A WOMAN'S LOT

1 **Introduction**   3
The Times, They Are A Changing **4** Moving Away from the Prescription Pad **6** The Best Way Forward **7**

2 **Cycles of Change**   8
The 'Curse' or a Blessing? **8** A New Stage of Life **13** Post-Menopause **14**

3 **Dance of the Hormones**   15
Blood Sugar **15** Stress Hormones **18** Stress Raises Blood Sugar Levels **19** Adrenal Glands Also Produce Sex Hormones **20** Reduce Stress Levels **20** Thyroid Hormones **21**

4 **Oestrogen Overload**   23
What Is Going On? **24** Sources of Excess Oestrogens **25** The Link Between Diet and Oestrogen Balance **29** Restoring the Balance **30**

PART TWO

7-POINT PLAN FOR HORMONE HEALTH

5 **'Rubbish In, Rubbish Out'**   35
Point 1, Eat Healthy Fats **36**
Point 2, Whole Carbohydrates Are Vital **40**
Point 3, Fibre Eliminates Hormones **42**
Point 4, Eat Foods Rich in Plant-Oestrogens **43**
Point 5, Hydrate Your Body **46**
Point 6, Eat Vitamin- and Mineral-Rich Foods **48**

Point 7, Exercise To Eliminate Oestrogens **50**
6 **Menu Plans** 52

PART THREE
REDUCE EXPOSURE

7 **Cut Out Chemicals** 61
Chemicals In Our Food **62** Cooking Utensils **63** Water Quality **63** Household Products **64** Personal Care **64**
8 **Pills and Patches** 65
The Contraceptive Pill **66** The Contraceptive Pill Affects Nutritional Status **69** Stopping the Pill **72** Progestogens – Not Progesterone by Another Name **73** HRT – Hormone Replacement Therapy **74** SERMs **75** Fertility Treatment **77**

PART FOUR
NATURAL HORMONES

9 **Phytohealth** 81
Sources of Phytoestrogens **82**
10 **Herbs for Harmony** 85
11 **Natural Hormones** 91
Natural Progesterone **91** How the Body Uses Progesterone **91** How to Use Natural Progesterone **92** What Is Natural About Taking Progesterone? **96** Natural Oestrogen **97** Find a Friendly GP **98** Testing Hormone Levels **98**

PART FIVE
TARGETING HEALTH

12 **Introduction** 103
13 **Balancing Blood Sugar Levels** 104

14	**Boosting Your Thyroid**	110
15	**Thrush and Cystitis**	112
16	**Moontime Madness**	117
	High Progesterone PMS 119 Heavy Periods 120 Period Cramps 122 Irregular Periods 123 Bloating 124 Diet to Banish PMS 125 Mood Swings 127	
17	**Fertility**	129
	Natural Family Planning 129 Preparing for a Healthy Pregnancy 130 Infertility 132 Healthy Sperm 133	
18	**Bosom Buddies**	135
	Healthy Breasts 137	
19	**What's Up Down Under**	139
	Fibroids 139 Endometriosis 140 Ovarian Cysts 143 Polycystic Ovaries 144 Pelvic Inflammatory Disease (PID) 145 Cervical Erosion and Dysplasia 146 Staying Away from the Surgeon's Knife 147 Cancers of the Reproductive Tract 149	
20	**Managing Your Menopause**	151
	Is Soya Natural HRT? 152 Cooling Hot Flushes 153 Exercise 154 Menopausal Weight Gain 154 A Healthy Heart 155 Remedies for Other Common Menopausal Problems 157 Progesterone and the Menopause 158	
21	**Reversing Osteoporosis**	159
	Risk Factors for Osteoporosis 161 Bone Building 162 Does Drinking Milk Help Osteoporosis? 163 Vitamin D 165 Beefing Up Your Bones? 166 Vitamin K 166 Low Stomach Acidity 167 Other Factors 168 The Lee Study 168	
22	**Closing Thoughts**	171

PART SIX

APPENDICES

Appendix I – Monthly Chart	174
Appendix II – Sources of Fibre	176
Resources	178

Herbal and Nutrient Supplement Supplies 178 To Find a Nutritional Therapist 179 Support Groups 180 Natural Family Planning and Preconception 180 Books 180 Recipe Books 181 Natural Progesterone Information/Supplies 181 Biochemical Testing 181 Organic Food Sources 182 Distilled Water Suppliers 182 Chemical-Free Cosmetics and Household Products 182

Part One
A WOMAN'S LOT

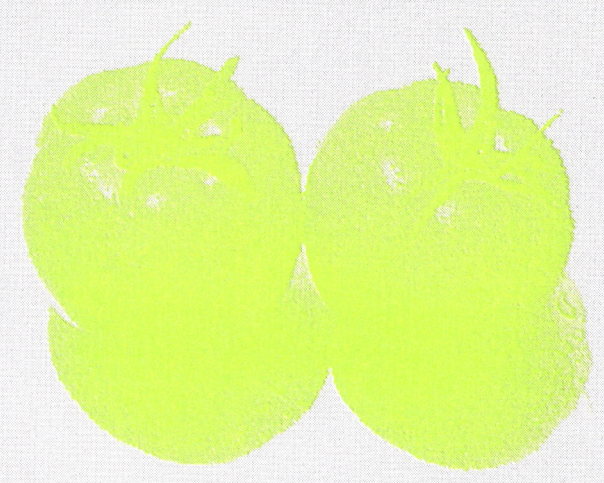

CHAPTER ONE

Introduction

Are women just meant to put up with their 'female problems'? Is it a woman's lot to go through a life overshadowed by premenstrual syndrome (PMS), fertility problems, menopausal symptoms, and possibly fibroids, endometriosis and other disorders? Of course not. Mother Nature did not design us to clutch a hot-water bottle to our abdomens every month, or to sweat all night as we come to the end of our reproductive life. She meant us to move reasonably easily through all these transitions.

One fact always surprises me when counselling women about their health. In a survey of the women who came to see me, only about ten per cent of them mentioned hormonal problems as a specific issue they wanted to address. And yet around 80 per cent of those women ticked boxes which were relevant to hormonal imbalance (such as PMS, menopausal problems or hysterectomies). The majority of women, when questioned, were not fully aware that anything could successfully be done about their cramps, bloated breasts, hot flushes or osteoporosis, yet these symptoms respond well to natural treatment, and dramatic improvements can be made, even in the most resistant cases, with a little perseverance.

The life cycle of a woman takes her through stages which are dominated by changes in her fertility – from the onset of menstruation as a young girl, through monthly cycles, possible pregnancy and breastfeeding, to the peri-menopause (pre-menopausal stage), menopause and the post-menopausal stage. All of these are natural phases which have been going on from time immemorial.

Now, in the early stages of the 21st century, we have reached a situation where we have increasing medicalisation of these natural phenomena. Social change, shifts in our diet, medical and pharmaceutical innovations and environmental hazards have all combined to alter women's hormonal health, as well as change the perspective on how such problems are viewed.

The changes in hormonal cycles which take place throughout a woman's life are now seen as steps which can be interrupted and manipulated. In the case of the menopause, it is common to treat it as a deficiency disease – a hormone or two are lacking so we simply replace them. This thinking is in line with other areas of health management where we have a strongly interventionist view of many diseases – if something doesn't work, medicate it, whip it out or replace it. We have seen great increases in the incidence of various symptoms and diseases but, rather than look at why these changes are happening, we try to manage them once they have occurred – and then not always successfully.

These days, four out of five women of child-bearing age suffer from PMS, one in ten have endometriosis and one in five who are investigated have ovarian cysts. Of huge concern is the fact that these diseases are also developing at earlier stages in women's lives. Fibroids, ovarian cysts and endometriosis were once rare in teenage girls, but are now commonly diagnosed and sadly they often result in permanent infertility.

THE TIMES, THEY ARE A CHANGING

Social changes, over the past 50 years or so, have been significant. In an earlier era, discussion of female 'problems', even amongst women, would not have been possible. Now many are happy to talk about all aspects of their reproductive history in frank detail and acres of shelf space are devoted to magazines and books which explore all the angles. This has led to a climate which questions the facilities available to women for the management of their hormonal health.

The effects of diet on menstruation are reasonably well known. It is fairly common knowledge that women who are malnourished, whether through famine or anorexia, experience late onset of, or interruptions in, their cycle. What is less well known is that the onset of periods in young women has steadily been getting earlier, with puberty moving from an average age of 14.5 at the beginning of the 20th century to an average age of 11 now. This is believed to be largely due to the impact of diet and physical activity. During a woman's life she will now have fewer pregnancies on average than previous generations. These two factors, earlier puberty and fewer pregnancies, have led to an increase in the number of menstrual cycles to which the average women is exposed, and therefore to the effects of female hormones on her body.

Diet is a key factor affecting hormone health, and our typical diet has changed dramatically in the last 50 years, with a greater dependence on processed, convenience foods. The type of food we eat can influence hormone processing in the body and encourage different 'pathways' for hormones to take. Depending on the route followed, the hormones can be damaging or benign. Certain foods, and the amount of exercise we do, can also determine whether hormones are eliminated successfully, or allowed to re-circulate – where they have the potential to cause mischief.

Another major change during this time has been our exposure to a vast array of chemicals in the environment. These chemicals come at us from all angles: the food we eat, the water we drink, the products we use in our homes and in our gardens. Hundreds of chemicals are being taken into our bodies to which we were not exposed only 50 years ago. And the bombshell which is only now moving into the public arena for discussion is that a significant number of these chemicals have the effect of altering female hormone balance.

The final change that has had an impact on our hormonal health is the availability of hormone drugs, including the contraceptive pill and HRT. These pills and patches have been promoted as the answer to all our prayers since they offer easy, trouble-free ways of manipulating our cycles to our advantage with almost no downsides. Or at least, if there are downsides, they can be deferred to another time of our lives – benefit now, pay later.

MOVING AWAY FROM THE PRESCRIPTION PAD

Women today are questioning the wisdom of turning to artificial measures to alleviate their 'female problems'. Often they are astounded to learn that symptoms such as hot flushes are not experienced to the same degree by women in other, non-Western, cultures who have different lifestyles and diets.

In the UK, prescriptions for hormone treatments have risen sharply in the last ten years, as more women have been made aware of the availability of hormone drugs. Daily reports in the media extol their virtues, and doctors prescribe them readily. Yet during this time a very significant number of women have elected to take another route to achieve hormonal balance in their lives. Women are now viewing imbalances in hormones, not as nuisances which need to be suppressed at all costs, but as a sign that all is not well and that balance must be restored to ensure the health of the whole woman.

Women are now seeking the root causes of their hormone imbalance. There is great interest in balancing the hormones in more natural and gentle ways – dietary manipulation, avoiding 'gender bender' hormones in the environment, and using herbal remedies which have been known for centuries to positively influence hormone balance.

THE BEST WAY FORWARD

The priority is to understand what the root causes of hormone imbalance are and to address these imbalances as naturally as possible. If you give your body the raw materials it needs, it will usually sort out how to achieve balance. Imbalance is a protest on the part of your body that it is not getting what it needs to do the job properly. It is an uphill battle sometimes, because we are surrounded with artificial chemicals, but for the most part diet, and judicious use of supplemental vitamins, minerals and herbs can be sufficient. In some cases, because hormone imbalance has gone too far, or because of a woman's genetic make-up, there may be a place for hormone replacement, but not as a first port of call. And those hormones serve us best if they are identical to those we manufacture in our bodies. All too often we employ the sledgehammer approach of pharmaceutical hormones that use alien 'look-alike' hormones. Even if the hormones are natural they must not be viewed as a 'pill for an ill' at the expense of getting diet and lifestyle factors right in the first place.

This book is aimed at examining the issues surrounding natural hormone balance for women who prefer to take a holistic view of their health and who plan to live many happy, healthy and fruitful years.

CHAPTER TWO

Cycles of Change

Understanding the ebb and flow of the two main female hormones, oestrogen and progesterone, is the first step in having a picture of how best to alleviate your particular hormone balance problems.

The female reproductive tract consists of the uterus (or womb), the cervix, the ovaries and the fallopian tubes. The lining of the uterus is called the endometrium. Every month, during a woman's reproductive years, these organs, with the aid of hormones, prepare for the arrival of a baby. The uterus is normally the size of a fist but it can stretch to accommodate a baby the size of a watermelon. The muscles of the uterus are unique in the body, and not only are they able to deliver the baby by their contractions, they are also able to return the uterus to its normal size within a few weeks of delivery.

The female hormones are produced principally by the ovaries with back-up hormones being produced by the adrenal glands and by fat cells. Hormone production is governed by the 'master glands', the hypothalamus and pituitary glands which are located within the brain.

THE CURSE OR A BLESSING?

At puberty, the female hormones are triggered into action, having previously been dormant. The trigger comes from the hypothalamus, which instructs the pituitary to release follicle stimulating hormone (FSH) and luteinising hormone (LH). Together these hormones stimulate the ovaries to mature and release an egg ready for fertilisation. The lining of the womb is thickened, but when the egg is not fertilised the lining is shed and this is the girl's first period.

It takes around three years, from onset, for the regularity of the cycle to become fully established. During a woman's reproductive life of around 40 years she will have a total of about 400 cycles. The number of periods she actually has is influenced by the number of pregnancies she has, whether she breast-feeds and the ages at which she starts her periods and has her menopause. In some cultures women may have as few as 100 periods during their lives as they have more pregnancies than women who live in the West, start their periods later and have earlier menopauses.

The First Half of The Cycle – Days 1-14

Menstruation happens approximately every 28 days, though it is not unusual for women to have differing cycles, spanning anything from 20 days to 40 days. For the sake of simplicity we will talk in terms of a 'normal' cycle.

At the start of the cycle levels of the two hormones, oestrogen and progesterone, are low and the lining of the uterus has just been shed. This happened because the egg was not fertilised. These low levels of hormones act as a trigger for the hypothalamus to start its job of stimulating the next egg to be released. It does this by producing FSH. FSH encourages a follicle in one of the ovaries to mature and ripen an egg. At the same time it also encourages oestrogen production by the ovaries to steadily increase. The job of oestrogens is to make the womb ready to receive the egg if it is fertilised. It causes the lining of the womb to thicken and breast tissue to become more active.

On around day 12, oestrogen levels peak and this triggers

another hormone from the hypothalamus, LH. On day 14 the surge of LH triggers the release of the mature egg from the follicle. The egg now starts its two- or three-day journey down the fallopian tube into the womb where, if it is fertilised, it is meant to implant itself and start the pregnancy.

The Second Half of The Cycle – Days 15-28

After the egg is released the space left behind by the ruptured follicle develops into a group of specialised cells, called the corpus luteum. The corpus luteum takes on the role of producing both oestrogen and progesterone. Both of these hormones are designed to prepare the woman's body to receive a fertilised egg. Progesterone is essential to maintain a pregnancy, which is implied by its name – PRO-GESTation. One of the effects of progesterone is to raise body temperature and many women will check to see when they ovulate, for family planning purposes, by checking their temperature in the middle of their cycle (see **Natural Family Planning** on page 129).

If an egg has been fertilised successfully the levels of these two hormones continue to increase steadily. If, however, the egg has not been fertilised, the corpus luteum begins to wither as it has no use. The destruction of the corpus luteum triggers a sharp fall in the two hormone levels, and this in turn causes the blood vessels supplying the lining of the uterus to go into spasm for it to be shed. The resulting low levels of hormones then act as a signal to the hypothalamus to secrete FSH, and the whole process begins again.

A Happy Event

If the egg is fertilised, the corpus luteum continues to produce oestrogen and progesterone in increasing amounts for the first

Hormone Changes During Menstruation

Day 1	Low oestrogen levels No progesterone	Lining of uterus previously shed Low hormone levels signal FSH to be secreted
	Oestrogen levels rise slowly	Egg ripens Lining of womb thickens
Day 12	Oestrogen levels peak	High oestrogen signals LH to be secreted
Day 14	LH surge	Triggers release of egg
	Oestrogen levels remain high. Progesterone levels rise	
Day 24	Oestrogen and progesterone levels fall	Lining of uterus shed (period)
Day 28	Last day of cycle	

trimester of the pregnancy, after which the placenta is able to take over this job.

Once the fertilised egg has successfully embedded in the womb on around the second or third day after its release, another hormone is produced called human chorionic gonadotrophic hormone (hCG). It is this hormone which is checked for in pregnancy tests.

The high levels of oestrogen and progesterone during a pregnancy mean that the feedback to the hypothalamus does not happen, and the release of FSH is suppressed. Oestrogen and progesterone levels will not fall again until the woman is ready to deliver the baby around nine months later. Different hormones bring about labour. The main delivery hormone, oxytocin, stimulates the womb to contract, and levels remain high until the baby is born. It also stimulates the delivery of the placenta, and nowadays oxytocin is injected immediately after delivery of the baby to speed up the delivery of the placenta.

After the baby is delivered, oestrogen levels will remain relatively low. Progesterone is not produced in significant amounts while the mother is breastfeeding and this creates a situation where a subsequently fertilised egg is unlikely to be promoted. This is why breastfeeding is sometimes viewed as a form of contraception, though it is not necessarily reliable.

Hormone Changes During Pregnancy

Day 14	LH surge	Triggers release of egg which is fertilised
Day 17	Oestrogen and progesterone levels continue to rise, hCG produced	The fertilised egg implants in uterus FSH and LH suppressed
3 Months	Placenta takes over job of producing oestrogen and progesterone	

A NEW STAGE OF LIFE

Strictly speaking, the term menopause means the time of a woman's final period. The 'change of life', as it is often called, is usually a ten-year period of hormonal changes which lead up to this moment, and is more accurately called the peri-menopause. On average, the process will start around the age of 45 and end at around 55, though a significant number of women, one in a 100, will have a very early menopause, which can occur at any time from their teens to their mid-thirties.

As oestrogen levels begin to decline with the peri-menopause, menstrual flow becomes lighter and sometimes more irregular, until it eventually stops completely. During the peri-menopause phase there are likely to be many menstrual cycles where an egg is not released at all and therefore progesterone is not produced either. These are called anovulatory cycles.

The drop in oestrogen levels signals the hypothalamus to secrete more FSH in an attempt to get the whole process of ovulation going again. Very few eggs are left at the time of the menopause for FSH to work on, and this means that the increase of FSH is in vain and levels eventually drop. By measuring FSH levels it may be possible to get an idea of which stage of the peri-menopause or menopause a woman is at. However, the ovaries do not just switch themselves off overnight, or even necessarily run themselves down smoothly. What happens more often is that they vacillate in their output, which can make measuring FSH unreliable. The limitation of the test is that it will just tell you what is going on on that particular day.

The ideal is that the change in hormone levels happens in a fairly smooth and steady way to ease the passage into this new stage of life. However, not all women experience an easy transition into menopause and we will talk about how to deal with this in **Managing Your Menopause** page 151.

Hormone Changes During the Peri-menopause

- Oestrogen levels gradually decline.
- Progesterone often produced erratically and only during cycles where an egg is released.
- Low oestrogen and progesterone levels encourage high FSH (leading to hot flushes).
- Levels of oestrogen eventually so low that menstruation ceases.

POST-MENOPAUSE

After periods stop, levels of oestrogen drop to around 40 per cent of their pre-menopausal levels as they continue to be produced by the adrenal glands and by fat cells. Progesterone is produced at very low levels by the adrenal glands – around 1 per cent of original levels. Many women view this time of hormonal quiescence as an opportunity to enjoy life unfettered by monthly cycles. Other women fear it as a loss of their youth. Low levels of hormones have been linked to an increase in the risk of a number of female, age-related health problems, including osteoporosis and heart disease, which, understandably, many women are keen to avoid. Hormone cancers such as breast cancer are also a greater risk post-menopausally. Examining the differences in incidence of these problems, and other hormone-related issues, between women on a Western diet and those on diets of other cultures gives many clues about how to prepare for and manage this stage successfully. In most Eastern countries, the incidence of these killer diseases is far below our own.

Hormone Levels Post-menopausally

Oestrogen produced at around 40 per cent of pre-menopausal levels, by the adrenal glands and by fat cells, and progesterone produced at around 1 per cent of pre-menopausal levels by the adrenal glands.

CHAPTER THREE

Dance of the Hormones

In order to achieve balanced female hormone health, it is not enough just to look at oestrogens and progesterone. There are a number of hormones which work together, to perform a balancing act, and if any of them are out of synchronism they will affect the others. This subtle relationship between the hormones means that achieving overall balance is probably the answer to many health issues. Hormones work on a feedback mechanism with many 'feedbacks' working in a pattern. This can best be imagined as a ballet or dance with interweaving circles, all of which affect each other. The hormones that are worth learning a little more about are the blood sugar hormones, the adrenal or stress hormones, and the thyroid hormone, thyroxine. The diagram overleaf helps to underscore the relationship between these hormones and the female hormones.

BLOOD SUGAR

Glucose is carried in our blood to all the cells in the body – and to the brain – for fuel. The level that glucose is at in the blood is called the blood sugar level, and we need to maintain a certain level for balanced energy. If our blood sugar goes too high, or too low, the body's hormonal systems interpret this as a crisis and the situation is rectified as a matter of urgency. The hormones which influence blood sugar levels are insulin, which

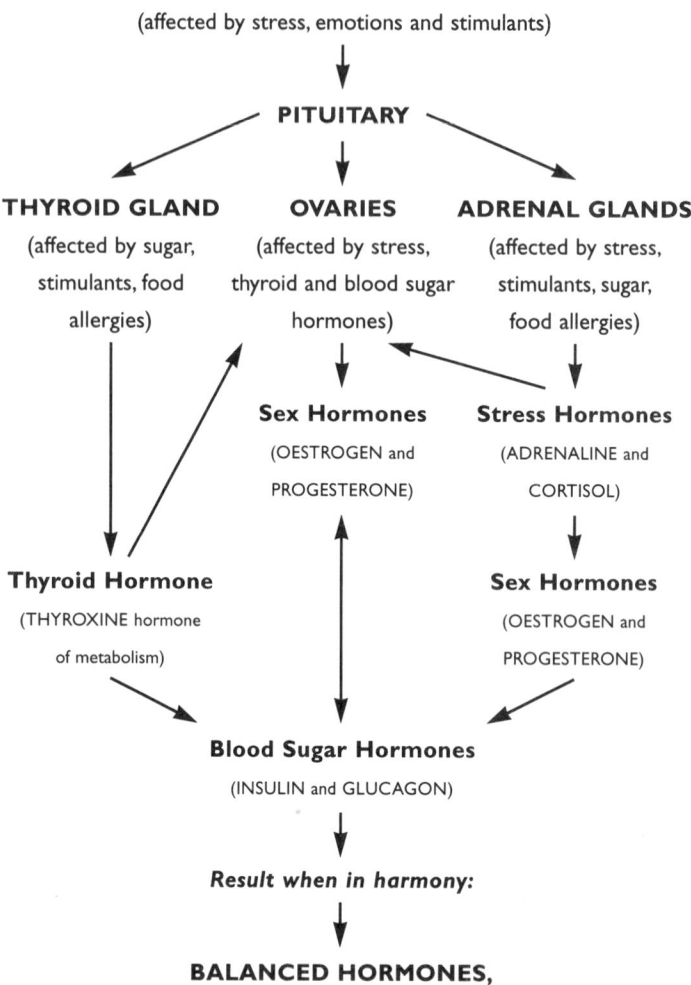

lowers a high blood sugar level, and glucagon, which raises blood sugar levels.

As hormones do not work in isolation, the effect that the female hormones can have on blood sugar regulation, and vice versa, is significant. Any woman who experiences the compulsion to eat sugary foods or to binge on foods in the few days before her period, which she would normally not be tempted to eat, will have a clear idea of how the hormones interact.

Insulin levels which are constantly being kept too high by a diet rich in sugars and refined carbohydrates can have a detrimental effect on female hormone health. Insulin encourages high levels of 'free' circulating oestrogens which, because they are not 'bound', allow them to do more damage to oestrogen-sensitive tissues such as breast tissue. This is likely to contribute to the problems of breast, and other hormonal, diseases.

The foods we eat have a direct effect on our blood sugar levels. We need to aim for a steady level of blood sugar which provides constant energy for our cells and brain. If you find that you are on a diet which repeatedly includes sugary foods, refined starches such as white bread or rice, or feel the need for stimulants as a 'pick-me-up', the chances are that you are experiencing blood sugar irregularities. In addition to foods there are other substances, and even activities, which trigger irregular blood sugar levels. Alcohol, caffeinated drinks and foods, stress, and even over-exercising can all stimulate high blood sugar levels. We will look at why this happens when we discuss stress in the following section.

Signs of imbalanced blood sugar levels include: low energy levels, drowsiness during the day, cravings for sweet foods, mood swings, anxiety and tension, insomnia, depression and addictions.

Recommendations to help regulate blood sugar levels are made in the chapter **Balancing Blood Sugar Levels** on page 104.

STRESS HORMONES

It is virtually impossible to live in our modern society without complaining about stress levels. They seem to be an occupational hazard of life. The stress response, called the 'fight or flight' response, evolved in days when we needed to deal with physical threats. If our ancestors were roaming the plains and came across a predator, the rush of adrenaline was designed to make them respond to the emergency by fighting the threat, or fleeing at top speed. Nowadays there are not so many predators around, but we get an idea of how powerful this response is when we are in a near-accident in the car and our foot goes to the brake instantly to avert disaster. In that moment your heart pounds, your pupils dilate, the hairs at the back of your neck stand up, your blood is diverted away from your digestive tract towards your skeletal muscles, your blood thickens in case of injury leading to the need for blood clotting, and so on . . . All these physical responses happen in an instant.

But of course in this day and age the need for this powerful reaction is rare. Yet stress of any sort results in this type of response to one degree or another – even if it is merely provoked by a row with the kids, or because you are late for work. This can lead, over time, to a wearing down of the body systems which deal with stress. Stress is related to digestive problems, cardiovascular problems, lowered immunity, muscle strains, and even cancer.

The adrenal glands produce our stress hormones, adrenaline and cortisol, and they are intimately affected by any chronic stresses on the body, whether these come in the form of external stress, emotional stress or dietary stress.

If the adrenal glands are either over-stimulated or fatigued – because of long-term chronic stress, disease or illness, a dependency on stimulants such as caffeine and alcohol, excess sugar over long periods of time or addiction to sensitivity-provoking foods – they will function sub-optimally and this can result in reduced capacity of these vital glands.

STRESS RAISES BLOOD SUGAR LEVELS

One of the main effects of adrenaline is to trigger the hormone glucagon, which is responsible for raising blood sugar levels by mobilising glycogen energy stores from the liver and the muscles. It does this because immediate blood sugar is needed to fuel the fight or flight response. However, if you are under constant stress, this means that your blood sugar is always being inappropriately triggered, and this can contribute significantly to blood sugar problems.

Stimulants, caffeine, recreational drugs, addictions (including, for instance, gambling and compulsive shopping) and over-exercising can all lead to this same response because all of these substances or activities trigger adrenaline, which in turn raises blood sugar levels. The knock-on effect on sex hormones is significant and the interaction between all of these hormones is particularly intimate. Another stress hormone, cortisol, when triggered to excess, has the detrimental effect of competing with progesterone. This means that progesterone is then unable to adequately fulfil one of its functions, which is balancing out oestrogen levels. High cortisol levels also have the effect of not allowing body tissues to regenerate and repair themselves.

ADRENAL GLANDS ALSO PRODUCE SEX HORMONES

Another important factor is that the adrenal glands, which produce these stress hormones, also have the function of producing some of the total oestrogen. If the adrenal glands have been over-exerted through a woman's life, they are unlikely to be as efficient as they might be at producing the female hormones. This has implications for the menopause, when the ovaries stop producing the female sex hormones. In normal circumstances it would be expected that the adrenal glands would carry on providing sufficient oestrogen to reduce the impact of menopausal problems. But in many women they are so adrenally-exhausted by the time they reach this stage of their lives that this function is not carried out efficiently.

REDUCE STRESS LEVELS

The key message is to nurture your adrenal glands by avoiding dietary stresses and stimulants such as sugar, alcohol, cigarettes, coffee or strong tea.

If you are adrenally-stressed, it is vital to support the recovery of the adrenal glands by addressing the stress in your life. We all know what areas of stress are major influences in our lives, and most of us also know what strategies we need to employ to deal with these. Often it is just a question of getting round to implementing them! Maybe it is now time to act by:

- Creating strategies if you do not already have them.
- Establishing what your goals are.
- Focussing on realistic steps and goals.
- Focussing on positive goals, not negative ones (i.e. 'I am a non-smoker', not 'I wish I didn't smoke').
- Doing more of what you enjoy.

- Learning to say no when you are tempted to say maybe.
- Taking time out each day for yourself.
- Taking holidays.
- Staying well by eating healthily. Illness is stressful, support your physical health.
- Act on what you can change and don't worry about what you can't change.

The main dietary support for adrenal stress is to follow the advice in **Balancing Blood Sugar Levels** on page 104, where suggestions are also made about additional supplements to support adrenal gland health.

THYROID HORMONES

The thyroid gland produces a hormone, thyroxine, which is the hormone responsible for metabolism and heat regulation. It governs the transfer of energy into every cell in the body, and this means that there are far-reaching consequences if the thyroid gland is not operating optimally. The thyroid, when it is not working efficiently, can be either underactive or overactive.

Signs of possible underactivity of the thyroid include:
excessive tiredness, a tendency to put on weight, oversensitivity to cold temperatures, bloating, blood sugar regulation problems, low blood pressure.

Signs of possible overactivity of the thyroid include:
elevated body temperature, a tendency to be underweight, a tendency to be hyperactive, 'bulging' eyes.

The relationship between an underactive thyroid and imbalanced sex hormones is stronger than for an overactive thyroid, and you can also see that many of the symptoms mirror oestrogen excess or premenstrual symptoms. An excess of oestrogens can depress thyroid hormone production. Progesterone can bolster the effects of the thyroid hormone. A good illustration of this is that women's temperatures elevate slightly at the time of ovulation when progesterone is being produced.

If you think that you may have an underactive thyroid, this can be checked easily by your doctor. If your thyroid is clinically under-functioning, your doctor will give you a prescription for thyroid hormone replacement. Sometimes it is not necessary to take the full dose, and you can take a slightly lower-dose to achieve the necessary results. This measure helps to reduce the risk of your body becoming dependent on supplementing the hormone – discuss this with your doctor.

It has been estimated that one in four women have an underactive thyroid, though this might not be bad enough to show up in laboratory tests. One way of telling if you have a possible underactive thyroid, if the test from your doctor proves negative, is to take your underarm temperature, for ten minutes, every day for a month, *before* you get out of bed. The idea is to take your temperature before you have raised your metabolism by getting up, even to go to the bathroom. You will need to remember to shake down the thermometer the night before and leave it on your bedside table. If, after a month, your averaged-out underarm temperature is below 36.5°C/97.8°F your thyroid may be operating sub-optimally. This is because the thyroid hormone is responsible for, amongst other things, keeping your temperature up to a normal level. If you find that your thyroid function might need supporting, follow the advice in **Boosting Your Thyroid** on page 110.

CHAPTER FOUR

Oestrogen Overload

There is an old Chinese curse 'May You Live In Interesting Times'. We currently live in 'Interesting Times' hormonally speaking, and here are some 'Interesting' hormonal facts to consider:

- Puberty in girls has become a much earlier event, with the average onset occuring nowadays at age 11 compared to age 14.5, 100 years ago. Early puberty exposes a woman to higher levels of oestrogens during her lifetime.
- According to two surveys conducted by the Women's Nutritional Advisory Service in 1985 and 1996, the severity of PMS symptoms is on the increase.
- The incidences of fibroids, ovarian cysts and endometriosis are all on the increase. Fibroids occur in four out of five women (though most do not get to the point where they cause problems). Ovarian cysts occur in one in five women examined, and endometriosis in one in ten women.
- The average sperm count has dropped by half in the last 50 years – a very short time span.
- The number of boys born with genital defects, called hypospadias, has doubled from one in 300 to one in 150.
- Since the 1960s there has been a 60 per cent increase in undescended testes. This can increase the risk of infertility and testicular cancer.
- According to a report by Macmillan Cancer Relief and Cambridge University in 1997, incidence of various hormone related cancers is set for massive increases over a

period of 30 years. From 1985 to 2015, breast cancer is set to rise by 52 per cent, cervical cancer by 7 per cent and uterine cancer by 83 per cent.
- Men are not immune to hormone influences, with prostate cancer set to rise by an astounding 234 per cent and testicular cancer by 50 per cent over the same period.
- Wildlife has been undergoing some disturbing disruptions to sexual development, mating behaviour and failing fertility. In the 1980s alligators in Lake Apopka were found to have shrunken genitalia, which led to a sharp drop in egg laying by females. Ranched minks fed fish from the Great Lakes fail to reproduce, while mink fed fish from other sources are fine. Four per cent of polar bears, in a sample of 2000, have been born with dual sex organs. Male Texan turtles are being born with ovaries. And these are only some of the examples.

WHAT IS GOING ON?

Why are these changes happening in such a short time span? There is one theory which seems to hold sway over all others, and which goes a long way to explaining these disturbing phenomena. We are living in interesting times indeed – we are living in times of oestrogen overload. Experts are saying that the unifying factor in all of these strange events is they are influenced by oestrogens in our environment, and by dietary factors which prevent us from excreting oestrogens efficiently. One of the main effects of oestrogen is to encourage plumping out of tissues and to speed up cell division. If oestrogen levels are high, these effects can result in, for example, bloating or breast cysts, or even female reproductive tract cancers. The effects on future generations are unquantified but it is feared that they may be dramatic. With lowered sperm counts, increased incidence of baby boys born with malformed genitals, and questions surrounding girls who are third-generation contraceptive pill users, it would appear that the cumulative effects of hormone disruption on future generations could be serious.

Oestrogen overload can lead to:
- Swollen breasts and discomfort premenstrually.
- Increased risk of endometriosis, ovarian cysts and fibroids.
- Lowered thyroid hormone effectiveness, contributing to feeling cold, bloated and having a sluggish metabolism.
- Significantly increased risk of breast cancer both pre- and post-menopausally. It also increases the risk of cervical and uterine (endometrial) cancer.
- In men, raised levels of environmental oestrogens are linked to an increased risk of prostate and testicular cancers.

It would be great to be able to say that if we eliminated our exposure to oestrogens from one source we could rectify the balance. But it is not like that, and our exposure comes from a number of sources.

Oestrogens are not all bad, and we will learn in later chapters about how healthy oestrogens can help to balance the equation. Plant oestrogens, for instance, can help to maintain bone density in later years and to reduce the risk of cardiovascular disease (see **Phytohealth** on page 81). However many oestrogens to which we are exposed are being found to have very worrying consequences, including all of the ones listed above.

SOURCES OF EXCESS OESTROGENS

Anovulatory cycles: Women, mostly from their mid-thirties onwards, have cycles when they do not produce an egg. During these cycles they will also not produce the progesterone hormone which is manufactured by the follicle left behind by the egg. This means that any oestrogens that they make, or to which they are exposed, will not be counter-balanced by progesterone, and as a result they can then have a magnified effect on the body. This is why some cycles can be worse than others with greater PMS symptoms.

Anovulatory cycles become greater in number before the menopause, and this can lead to oestrogen becoming increasingly dominant in women's bodies. One of the effects of this may well be the high proportion of breast cancers that are diagnosed in the ten years after the menopause. It takes several years for breast cancer to develop and a large number of cases probably have their roots in the earlier years when anovulatory cycles were being experienced.

Contributing factors to a woman's likelihood of having anovulatory cycles include nutrient deficiencies, stress and over-exercising.

Oestrogens not processed properly: There are three main oestrogens produced in our bodies. These are E1, E2 and E3 (oestrone, oestradiol and oestriol). The first two, E1 and E2, are 'strong' oestrogens and they are capable of having a detrimental effect if they are produced to excess, or if they cannot be eliminated. They are also capable of being partially converted into E3, which is a benign form of the hormone produced mostly when we are pregnant. Because E3 is a much less potent form of oestrogen it does not have the same potential downsides of the other two main forms. If our diets are insufficient to help balance hormones, then susceptible women will process oestrogens inappropriately. Additionally, a diet which is low in fibre will encourage oestrogens to be recirculated, rather than eliminated as they should be. This means that they are available to cause symptoms of oestrogen excess.

Hormone drugs: The oestrogens found in the contraceptive pill and in HRT are the type which have been found to be related to increased risk of hormone cancers. These oestrogens are mainly oestradiol and oestrone, and their association with female cancers is the same whether they come from the Pill or HRT, or if they are made in the body.

Environmental oestrogens: The most worrying oestrogens are environmental oestrogens, called xenoestrogens. A number of chemicals and products have been found to have strong oestrogenic characteristics. It seems we have entered into a Faustian pact. We enjoy all the benefits of our modern society by taking advantage of, for example, plastics, pesticides and household detergents, but at the significant price of disrupted hormone health.

When we eat these chemicals, or are exposed to them, our xenoestrogen load is increased. Governments of different countries have differing views about these chemicals. For instance, the acceptable daily intake of dioxins in the US is set at 0.0064 units, the World Health Organisation has set a figure of 1.4 units, while in the UK a level of 10 units is deemed acceptable. Another example is the pesticide Lindane, implicated in female hormonal cancers, which has been banned in a number of countries such as New Zealand, Sweden, Finland and the Netherlands. Other countries, such as the US, have classified it as a probable human carcinogen since the 1970s, but it is still permitted in the UK.

Animals are near the top of the 'food chain'. This means that foods they have eaten, which have been burdened with chemical oestrogens, concentrate in their fats. When we eat animal fats, we are exposed to these hormone-like chemicals.

Sources of xenoestrogens include:
- Pesticides, insecticides, herbicides, wood treatments, head lice treatments.
- Plastics, including chewable children's toys, cling film food wrap, plastic linings to cartons and tins.
- Industrial and farming compounds which find their way into the water supply.
- Foods such as sprayed vegetables and fruit, also meat, fish and dairy foods.

The oestrogens found from these external sources are not precisely the same as the oestrogens which we find in our bodies, but are close chemical relatives. They can best be described as hormone-mimickers and these uninvited guests are particularly disruptive. They are considerably stronger in effect when compared to our natural oestrogens, and also persist and build up in our body tissues.

The cumulative effect of all this exposure is to put people, both women and men, into a hyper-oestrogenic state. This means that we have more circulating oestrogens which can disrupt the normal workings of our body.

In addition to oestrogen overload there is also an issue relating to 'unopposed oestrogens'. This refers to the fact that, during a woman's fertile years, oestrogens and progesterone normally achieve a balance. When women have low progesterone levels, it is less easy for them to stabilise the oestrogens they produce, or are exposed to. Many medical practitioners with a leaning towards addressing hormone imbalance as naturally as possible, are finding that oestrogen overload can be dealt with, and harmony restored, by addressing diet, vitamin, mineral and herbal supplementation and, if symptoms then persist, by prescribing natural progesterone, which is discussed later in the book.

THE LINK BETWEEN DIET AND OESTROGEN BALANCE

The equilibrium of female hormones is influenced by dietary factors such as fat and alcohol intake, sugar balance and fibre levels.

Excessive amounts of fat in the diet encourage high oestrogen levels: body fat produces oestrogens in its own right; animal fats, and especially dairy products, come with their own oestrogen load from the animal; vegetable fats are rich sources of chemical oestrogen 'mimickers' in the form of pesticides. These three sources of oestrogens can add up if the overall diet is high in fats.

The effect of dietary fibre on oestrogens is well known, and is of paramount importance in regulating premenstrual problems. Fibre, which we tend to think of as a digestive aid, is so powerful a hormone modulator that it can reduce the risk of oestrogen-related breast cancer. If it can do that for breast cancer, imagine what it can do for other symptoms of oestrogen overload, including PMS, bloating and breast symptoms. Fibre acts as a sponge soaking up oestrogens and excreting them from the bowels, and up to 36 per cent fewer of the harmful oestrogens have been measured in the blood of women with high-fibre diets. The bowels are the normal route of excretion for oestrogens. If there is insufficient fibre, and transit time in the digestive tract is slowed down, the oestrogens have the time to be reabsorbed into the bloodstream, to recirculate, and to contribute to oestrogen-related bloating.

As we have already discussed, blood sugar balance which is out of synch because of excessive consumption of sugar, alcohol and other stimulants such as tea or coffee, can significantly affect female hormone balance, as well as thyroid and adrenal hormones. High insulin levels also serve to magnify the effects of oestrogens circulating in the blood.

The other critical link between oestrogen balance and diet is the liver. The liver is an organ to respect once you realise it has at least 40 different roles to play in maintaining health. Some of these relate to maintaining hormone balance, and because the liver is also an organ of digestion, digestive health is directly linked to hormone health. There is a vicious cycle of compromised digestion affecting liver function, which in turn leads to hormone imbalance. Oestrogens which are no longer required are broken down in the liver, but if the liver is overburdened or working sub-optimally, oestrogen breakdown is impaired, which means that oestrogen levels in the body remain high and in turn lead to symptoms of hormone imbalance. Liver health is affected primarily by the types of fats we eat, our alcohol and caffeine intake, and exposure to pollutants.

RESTORING THE BALANCE

There are three ways in which we can seek to restore hormone balance in the face of this onslaught. By breaking it down into these three key steps it makes it easier to see that it is not a hopeless battle against invisible foes! The guiding principles for re-establishing hormonal health are:

1. Give your body the chance to process oestrogens in a healthy way and to eliminate unhelpful oestrogens efficiently. The 7-POINT PLAN FOR HORMONE HEALTH in the next chapter is designed to help achieve this goal.
2. Reduce exposure to environmental oestrogenic chemicals as much as possible.
3. Give a helping hand to hormone health by using natural sources of plant hormones from foods, supplements and, if necessary, natural hormone preparations.

What follows in this book are three sections which discuss each of these key steps in detail. Finally, we will close with a section looking at specific female complaints, such as premenstrual problems, diseases of the womb and the menopause.

Part Two

7-POINT PLAN FOR HORMONE HEALTH

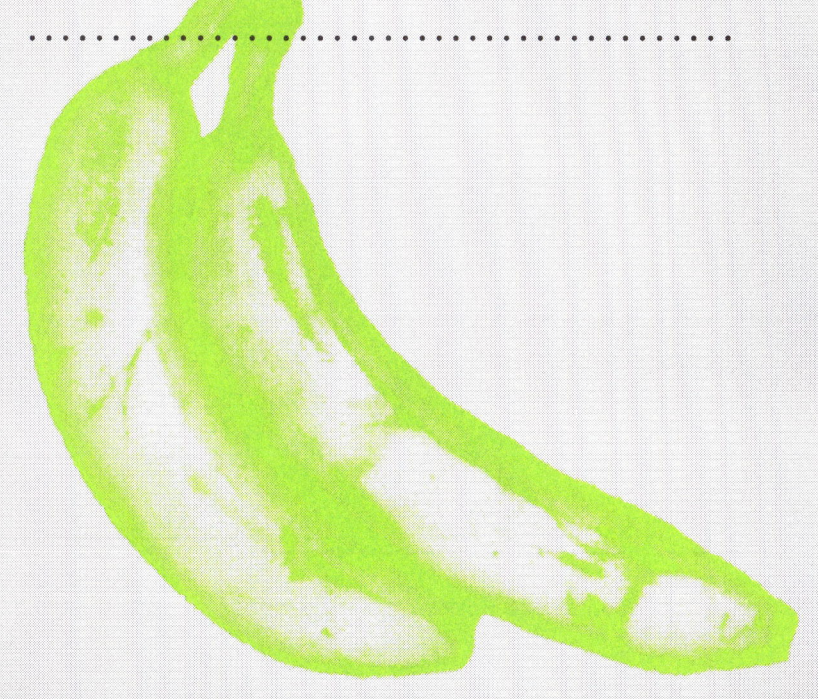

CHAPTER FIVE

'Rubbish in, rubbish out'

The foundation of health is the food you eat. To use computer terminology: Rubbish in, Rubbish out! If you eat in a way which conflicts with your body's needs, eventually it will rebel and symptoms will make themselves apparent. Hormone imbalance is one such symptom and it is an alarming indictment of the typical Western diet that so many women are subject to hormone health irregularities.

The food choices we make on a daily basis can make a real difference, helping to eliminate problems such as feeling wretched each month, experiencing menopausal symptoms, or being subjected to the more serious consequences of hormone imbalance such as fibroids, endometriosis, osteoporosis, or even breast, ovarian, cervical and endometrial cancers.

The following seven changes you can make will give you the best opportunity to regulate your hormones and bring your body into balance. Here is a summary:

POINT 1	Eat healthy fats
POINT 2	Whole carbohydrates are vital
POINT 3	Fibre eliminates hormones
POINT 4	Eat foods rich in plant-oestrogens
POINT 5	Hydrate your body
POINT 6	Eat vitamin- and mineral-rich foods
POINT 7	Exercise to balance hormones

One of the main aims of this eating programme is to encourage the body to process the three main oestrogens properly. Additionally, by balancing out blood sugar levels the negative impact of oestrogens is curtailed. Insulin produced when blood sugar levels are too high permits 'free' oestrogens to latch onto sensitive cells, such as those in the breast tissue, and amplify their activity. For more information about this see page 104 in **Balancing Blood Sugar Levels**. Finally, this plan improves bowel function, which allows the surplus oestrogens to be worked on by the bacteria in the bowels and to be eliminated correctly.

If your health concerns are about the menopause and a deficiency of oestrogens, then the plan is just as appropriate. Many of the foods discussed have the dual effect of countering oestrogens where there is an excess, but also providing gentle plant oestrogens where there is a deficiency. The most important foods for this are the grains, linseeds, soya foods and legumes (beans, pulses, peas, etc).

POINT 1: EAT HEALTHY FATS

Fats affect hormone balance in a number of ways. First and foremost the sex hormones are actually made from fats, so it is important to have them in the diet. This is why overly-restricted diets that exclude most fats, such as the type of diet that someone may follow if fasting for weight loss, can result in periods stopping – there literally isn't enough fat to make the hormones. On the other hand, too much fat is just as much of a problem. An excess of calories from fat has been linked to a variety of hormone health problems, especially female cancers. Fats are also major sources of environmental hormones obtained from our diet. Because of all of these factors it is important to get the right type and the right balance of fats in our diet. The fats in our diet are one of the main ways that environmental oestrogens are carried into our bodies. This includes the waxy coating on some fruits which trap chemicals, as well as oils, margarines and animal fats. Fats are high in calories and an excess of them predisposes us to putting on weight. Because our own fat cells also manufacture oestrogens this means that overweight people are likely to have an increased oestrogen output from their own fat cells.

Unhelpful fats: Two types of fats are likely to add to the problems of hormone imbalance, especially if they are eaten to the exclusion of the helpful fats. These are saturated fats found in meat and dairy products, and hydrogenated fats found in margarines and processed, packaged foods such as crisps, pies, biscuits and cakes. We do not really need to eat saturated fats at all as our body is very capable of making them, when needed, from starches and sugars in our diet, and hydrogenated fats can be positively harmful. Both of these types of fat increase the likelihood of inflammation, which is a feature of many hormone health problems such as swollen breasts, endometriosis and ovarian cysts. Hydrogenated fats have also been found in raised levels in the breast tissue of women with breast cancer.

Helpful fats: Two types of fats are healthy. These are monounsaturated fats, which are found mainly in olive oil, and polyunsaturated fats, found in oily fish, nuts, seeds, vegetables and their oils. The polyunsaturated fats help hormone health problems by having an anti-inflammatory effect on the body. This is why evening primrose oil has found such favour as treatment for premenstrual problems, and is even available on prescription from your doctor.

The helpful fats need careful handling as they are easily

destroyed by heat, light and long-term storage. Because of this seeds, nuts and oils such as sunflower or walnut oil are best bought in small quantities and kept in the fridge until their use-by date.

Steps to take

- Use virgin olive oil for cooking as it is more stable than other oils and is rich in antioxidants. These beneficial compounds, found in fruits and vegetables, such as olives, neutralise oxidation which is linked to inflammation, heart disease and cancer.
- Mix flax seeds in a glass jar with hemp, sunflower, linseed, pumpkin and sesame seeds in equal portions. Take out one heaped tablespoon daily and freshly grind. Added to cereals, yoghurts, soups or shakes they give a delicious flavour, as well as being powerhouses of minerals and healthy fats. You can munch on sunflower and pumpkin seeds for snacks.
- Add one tablespoon of cold-pressed polyunsaturated oils to your salads daily. Choose from cold-pressed flax, walnut, pumpkin, sesame or sunflower oils. These oils go rancid easily, so to get maximum benefit from them buy them in small bottles, made from dark glass, keep them in the fridge and use them within eight weeks of opening.
- Eat three portions of oily fish a week. The best choices are mackerel, sardines, salmon, anchovies, pilchards, eel, pink trout, shark or tuna. (Canned fish is fine, except for tuna which, during canning, is rendered low in helpful fats. See note about xenoestrogens from the lining of cans on page 63 in **Cut Out Chemicals**.) There is some concern about the dioxin levels found in fish, however the current state of knowledge suggests that the health benefits associated with

oily fish intake outweigh the risks attached to dioxin intake. It is also likely that cooked fish loses quite a lot of the dioxins accumulated.
- Spread choices to use instead of butter: mackerel paté, mushroom paté, tapenada, hummus, tahini, almond or other nut or seed butters.
- Limit fat from meat and dairy sources by trimming visible fat, choosing low-fat versions and limiting yourself to one portion of each daily. Choose leaner meat options such as skinless fish, skinless chicken or turkey, and game.
- Avoid hydrogenated fats in margarines and processed foods. Also avoid cooking with sunflower, corn or oils other than olive oil or coconut butter, if you can get it (none of these are significantly damaged by gentle heating). You can also use butter for cooking as it is also heat stable, however olive oil and coconut butter are healthier options.
- Cook by steaming, stir-frying or baking, and do not fry or eat burnt fatty foods. High temperatures change the nature of fats and create harmful carcinogenic (cancer-triggering) compounds.
- The quantity of fat is nearly as important as the quality of fats. We get an average of 40–45 per cent calories from fats, while the recommended amounts are a maximum of 30 per cent. This means that a woman eating 2000 calories daily should ideally have around 70 grams of fat per day. You can check food packages to see how many grams of fat they give per portion.

Healthy fats in supplements: Ideally you need to get good quality fats in the diet. Fats are macro-nutrients which we need in large quantities when compared to the micro-nutrients (vitamins and minerals). However, it can sometimes be useful to use supplements therapeutically for a while. For instance GLA, which is a type of fat found in evening primrose oil, starflower oil and borage oil, is extremely helpful for hormonal conditions such as PMS and hot flushes. Other sources of useful fats from supplements include fish oil capsules and flax oil capsules. These give different types of fats, EPA/DHA from fish oil and linolenic acid from flax oil. These are useful for conditions such as inflammation, heart disease, breast cancer and arthritis. Skin conditions also benefit hugely from both types of fats. Cod liver oil is best avoided these days as the livers of fish tend to be very polluted, as a result of which recent Government advice has been to avoid using liver oils for children. This does not affect the use of fish oil capsules extracted from fish flesh.

POINT 2: WHOLE CARBOHYDRATES ARE VITAL

The type of carbohydrates we eat are vital for maintaining blood sugar balance, and this in turn is vital for keeping our female hormones in check.

To put it simply there are two main types of carbohydrate:

- Whole, or complex carbohydrates, which have all their original fibre intact and break down slowly into sugar in the blood. This means that they are useful for maintaining a regular blood sugar balance and energy levels are kept constant.
- Refined, or simple, carbohydrates, which are either sugars or break down quickly into sugars in the blood. This means that they give a 'quick hit' of energy which feels good in the short-term, but peters out quickly, leaving you feeling low again. Refined foods are also intrinsically low in nutrients. For instance, wholewheat when turned into white flour is stripped of between 60–90 per cent of minerals such as calcium, magnesium, iron, zinc and chromium.

Another way of looking at this is that complex carbohydrates are brown and green foods, while refined carbohydrates are white foods. The more you can make selections from the list of complex carbohydrates, and reduce your intake of refined carbohydrates, the better your energy levels are likely to be. Balanced blood sugar will have a knock on effect and positively influence your hormonal balance.

Complex Carbohydrates	Simple Carbohydrates
(Brown and Green Foods) Lower in sugars, higher in nutrients	**(White Foods)** Higher in sugars, lower in nutrients
Wholemeal bread	White or 'brown' bread (not wh/m)
Brown rice	White rice
Brown pasta	White pasta (though still high in fibre)
Porridge oats	Instant oats
Muesli, bran cereals	Cornflakes, rice puffs
Oatcakes, rye crackers	Water biscuits
Jacket potato	Mashed/boiled potato (no skin)
Sweet potato	Most cakes and biscuits
Raw carrot, beets	Cooked carrots, parsnips, beets
Vegetables, salads	Sugar
Fruit (technically sugars, but have fibre)	Alcohol

POINT 3: FIBRE ELIMINATES HORMONES

Bowel health is intimately linked to hormone health, and fibre intake is essential to ensure healthy bowel movements. Women on higher fibre diets, such as vegetarians, have considerably lower levels of oestrogens circulating in their blood. Fibre also helps to regulate blood sugar levels which can help with premenstrual cravings. Pretty much all the authorities now agree that fibre levels in the diet, as well as being crucially linked to bowel disorders such as constipation, irritable bowel syndrome and even bowel cancer, are also linked directly to the incidence of hormone-related cancers such as breast and prostate cancers. There is also clear evidence that high-fibre diets significantly reduce other hormonal problems such as premenstrual problems. We eat, on average, around 9–10 grams of fibre daily, while the authorities recommend that we double this to at least 18 grams of fibre. Other experts, such as the National Cancer Institute in the US, recommend even higher levels of around 25–35 grams of fibre daily. For a breakdown of fibre levels in different foods see Appendix II on page 176. Simply put, if we include at least four pieces of fruit, a bowl of muesli or porridge, a couple of slices of wholemeal bread and a generous portion of beans, peas or lentils in our diet daily we should reach the 25–35 gram level. You can increase fibre in your diet by following these points:

- Legumes such as beans, peas, pulses, lentils, chick peas are rich sources of fibre. You can easily incorporate 1/2 to 1 cup of legumes daily in your diet by eating: lentil soup, bean salads, baked beans, green peas, hummus, Mexican bean dishes, bean curries. Use beans to bulk out pie dishes, to make soups or dips, or serve them as a vegetable side dish, or add to salads and stir-frys.
- Wholegrains are fibre-rich. It is therefore better to eat

porridge or muesli instead of rice puffs or cornflakes for breakfast, to use wholemeal or pumpernickel bread for sandwiches, buckwheat or wholewheat noodles, and brown rice for stir-frys, salads or for stuffing vegetables. These daily choices can make an important difference in boosting your fibre levels.
- Fruits and vegetables are essential to a fibre-rich diet. Eat a minimum of five portions a day – seven is better. Some fruit and vegetables have more fibre than others. The best include: pears, raspberries, figs, prunes, bananas, dried apricots, dates, mango, guava, gooseberries, plums, olives, loganberries, sweet potato, peas (a legume), plantain, yam and cabbage. Nuts, seeds and coconuts are also valuable sources of fibre.
- One quick way to increase fibre in your diet is to use added fibre. Wheat bran is too harsh for many people, and is also high in phytates which reduce the uptake of nutrients. More gentle fibre options to use include: oat fibre, rice fibre, freshly ground linseeds, psyllium husks and a type of sugar called FOS (fructo-oligo-saccharides). Beware of using too much added fibre of any type too quickly, especially if you have digestive problems, as it can make you windy and bloated. In this case introduce the added fibre very slowly to build up the tolerance of your digestive tract.

POINT 4: EAT FOODS RICH IN PLANT-OESTROGENS

Eating plant-oestrogens is a powerful tool for balancing hormones as they provide gentle forms of oestrogens which our bodies can use to advantage – either by boosting our supplies if needed at menopause and post-menopausally, or by opposing damaging oestrogens which may be sending our levels too high. This is just a brief introduction to this topic, and we discuss the subject of plant foods which are rich in hormones in more detail in the chapter **Phytohealth** on page 81. The best sources of plant-oestrogens are:

- Soya foods are the most concentrated sources. Ways of incorporating soya include:

  - Cooking soya beans in the same way as other beans and adding them to stews, casseroles, salads and soups, and using them to make dips.
  - Using soya milk instead of cows' milk for cooking, with cereals, and in desserts and drinks.
  - Eating soya yoghurts and using soya cheese for cooking.
  - Adding soya flour to baking recipes at a ratio of three parts 'normal' flour to one part soya flour.
  - Including soya flakes in a variety of dishes, for example adding them to breakfast cereals, or eating them as snacks (they have a nutty flavour).
  - Tofu can be added to a number of dishes. Use marinated tofu for kebabs and stir-frys, or mash plain tofu into dishes such as cottage pie or use as a stuffing for peppers. Alternatively, whizz plain tofu in a blender with soft fruit and soya milk for a creamy milk shake.
  - A number of soya and linseed 'muesli' bars are now becoming available. Breakfast cereals which include soya are likely to follow soon.
  - Breads are now widely available in supermarkets which are sometimes called 'Ladies' Breads'. They have linseeds and soya as main ingredients and they are particularly delicious and nutty in flavour.

This does not have to be a daunting programme. For instance, if you aim to have a portion of soya five times a week you might do the following:

Day 1   Have a soya yoghurt as a dessert
Day 2   Add soya flakes to morning cereal
Day 3   Eat a soya muesli bar as a snack
Day 4   Have soya milk on your cereal and in hot drinks
Day 5   Have a stir-fry for your evening meal with added tofu

- Linseeds, also called flax seeds, are fabulous sources of highly beneficial lignans, which are a type of plant-oestrogen. One or two tablespoons daily, added to cereals, yoghurts, shakes, soups, salads, baked goods or stews, can make a great difference to hormone balance. Build up to this level slowly from 1/4 tablespoon, and you will also find that they have a remarkably helpful effect on your bowels.
- All the legumes, and particularly chick peas, are very rich sources of plant-oestrogens. Chick peas can be made into hummus, curried, sautéed with onions and potato, or added to stews and roast vegetables.
- Wholegrains, in particular wholewheat and rye, are sufficiently strong in plant-oestrogen content to have successfully improved menopausal symptoms such as hot flushes in trials.
- Sprouted seeds such as alfalfa and sprouted soya beans or chick peas are excellent sources of plant-oestrogens and can be added to salads as fresh tasting and interesting ingredients.

POINT 5: HYDRATE YOUR BODY

One of the possible effects of hormone imbalance is water retention and bloating. An important strategy when dealing with this, and for general health, is to allow your system to flush itself out successfully and to stop body tissues becoming waterlogged. Our bodies are around 70 per cent water and we need two litres a day to replenish water lost and to keep our organs, especially our liver and kidneys which are responsible for detoxification, in good working order. The point at which you feel thirsty is already too late, and it means that you are already dehydrated internally. It is best to sip at drinks throughout the day, by keeping a water bottle or glass of water handy at all times. To hydrate your body:

- Drink plain water. As soon as water is mixed with anything else, it becomes more difficult for your body to process it. Getting the water drinking habit is one of the most important health tricks you can learn. Water quality is also important and it is a good idea to filter your water or to use good quality mineral water (spring water is not regulated in the same way as mineral water).
- After water the next best hydrating drinks, which are all excellent options include: fruit and herbal teas – some to try include rosehip, ginger and lemon, mint, blackcurrant – Rooibos tea, green tea, hot water with honey and lemon, fruit juice mixed at least 50/50 with plain water, sparkling water, juice as a hot drink with boiling water and pre-made spiced herbal drinks (available from health food shops).
- Avoid dehydrating drinks. Caffeine and alcohol are dehydrating and cause a net loss of water from the body, so satisfying your thirst with these drinks does not work in the long run. Caffeine is contained in coffee, teas, colas, chocolate, the herb guarana and some cold remedies and headache medicines. Caffeinated drinks to cut out include

coffee, strong tea and colas. Weak black tea has caffeine in it, but if you only drink it three or four times a day it should be fine, and you can benefit from the antioxidants in it. Caffeine is frequently implicated in breast pain and breast lumpiness premenstrually.

- Cut back on salt as this can worsen water retention. Most salt is eaten in processed foods, so limit these as well as avoiding the salt shaker. Instead of salt, use specially prepared seaweed in your grinder, low-salt foods and potassium salt substitutes.

- If water retention remains a problem you may need to address the possibility of food sensitivities. The most common foods to contribute to this problem are wheat, other grains such as oats or rye, dairy products and sometimes even soya.

- Moderate your alcohol intake as it is dehydrating. A major downside of alcohol is that it enhances oestrogen levels, which means that it is disruptive if you need to balance out your hormones – limiting yourself to four measures a week, or less, is the best plan. One of the clearest links between diet and oestrogen levels is alcohol. We are used to hearing about moderate levels of alcohol in a positive light as it has been linked to a reduction in cardiovascular risk. However, the research was conducted on men, precisely because of women's varying hormonal levels. What the results of the cardiovascular research fail to make clear is that even small amounts of alcohol, for example one unit a day, can magnify the effects of oestrogens in women. This means that any cardiovascular benefit may be outweighed by a detrimental effect on hormone problems, including breast and ovarian cancers. Post-menopausally, when women's hormone profiles are closer to men's, there may be a bit more leeway for a daily tipple of one measure.

POINT 6: EAT VITAMIN- AND MINERAL-RICH FOODS

Vitamins and minerals are the cogs in the wheels which keep all our functions running smoothly. Energy production, metabolism, hormone production, detoxification, mental processes and the functioning of every organ are all vitamin and mineral dependent. While supplements can help to keep us in optimal health, they are no substitute for a wide range of vitamins and minerals being derived from the diet. To make sure you do not fall short, remember these pointers:

- Eat a varied diet, in order to get a wide range of nutrients. If we are too restricted in our food choices we do not give our bodies the choice of all the nutrients which might be needed. For instance, as an alternative to wheat you could try the following grains:
  - oats (porridge, oatcakes, oat muesli, flapjacks)
  - corn (tortillas, corn chips, popcorn, pasta)
  - rye (crackers, bread)
  - millet (porridge, muesli flakes)
  - buckwheat (noodles, blini pancakes, kasha, pasta)
  - rice (rice cakes, noodles, pasta)
  - quinoa
  - barley
- Fruits and vegetables are by far the most valuable source of vitamins and minerals. The fresher the foods, the better the vitamin content is likely to be, and sometimes frozen vegetables may actually be better sources of vitamins than shop-weary greens. Eat at least three servings of fruit a day, and three servings of vegetables (dark green leafy, root, salad stuffs, the onion family or red/yellow/orange/purple vegetables).
- Mineral-rich sources also include legumes, whole grains,

fresh nuts and fresh seeds (for calcium, magnesium and zinc), eggs, small quantities of meat (for iron, zinc and some B vitamins), sardines and salmon (for calcium), and small amounts of dairy produce (yoghurt and cottage cheese are better options than cheese or milk).
- Cooking methods can help to preserve vitamins and minerals. Avoid boiling in water as minerals are lost to the cooking water – steam instead – and avoid cooking vegetables for longer than necessary to preserve vitamin content – vegetables which are still slightly crisp, or 'al-dente', are better than a soft texture. Stir-frying for short amounts of time retains many nutrients.

Vitamin and mineral supplements: How many vitamins and minerals you manage to absorb from your food depends not only upon making wise food choices, but also on other factors:

- Cooking methods that do not leach nutrients out of foods.
- A healthy digestion which is capable of making full use of the nutrients in foods.
- The conditions in which the foods were cultivated – foods are often grown in nutrient-depleted soil.
- The methods of transport, storage and preservation of foods.
- Nutrients are likely to be used up in greater quantities if you are under stress for an extended period of time.

It is best to get all the nutrients you need from your diet, however it can only help to take a good quality vitamin and mineral supplement. If you want to achieve doses which are useful, you will probably find that most of the once-a-day supplements which are sold inexpensively in supermarkets and chain stores do not fit the bill. Frankly, you usually get what you pay for with supplements. Good quality brands are significantly more absorbable, and can be used more efficiently by the body than their cheaper counterparts. The most important nutrients for managing hormones are magnesium (300–600 mg daily), calcium (250–500 mg daily), zinc 15–25 mg daily, chromium 200–500 mcg daily and B-complex (50–100 mg daily).

POINT 7: EXERCISE TO ELIMINATE OESTROGENS

The evidence is quite clear that exercise helps to regulate oestrogens in the body. Girls who exercise from a young age tend to have later onset of periods, which exposes them to less menstrual cycles, and therefore protects them to a degree from some of the harmful effects of long-term exposure to oestrogens. Menopausal symptoms are significantly less disruptive in those who exercise regularly when compared to those who do not. Women who exercise for four hours a week have a 37 per cent reduced risk of breast cancer because exercise limits oestrogen levels. One of the reasons why rural women in China and Japan do not experience the same set of hormone problems that we do in the West could be that they spend so much more time in physical labour. Lack of exercise could also partly explain the increase of hormone diseases in the West, since the 20th century has seen a significant decline in more labour-intensive jobs. Of course I'm not suggesting you go out to work in the fields or start hand-scrubbing your doorstep, though these might help! Even two hours a week of exercise is beneficial, though more quantifiable benefit seems to be achieved with four hours. On the other hand, overexercising is not helpful and again this can lead to disruption of menstruation.

- Choose an activity you enjoy – you are more likely to stick to it.

- Make an appointment with a friend – a tennis game or meet at a pool – again you are more likely to stick to it if you do not wish to let your friend down.
- Don't make grand plans that are unrealistic and may cause joint or muscle damage. Start slowly, with your doctor's approval if you have a pre-existing heart condition, and build up the amount of time and intensity over a period of a few weeks.
- Exercise to the point where your pulse is raised and you feel slightly breathless, but not to an intensity where you cannot hold a conversation.
- Always warm up first by doing some limbering exercises.
- Remember than exercise need not mean slogging it out on the treadmill at the local gym. Increasing activity levels in all ways is valid. Walking up stairs, instead of using the lift, a brisk walk, carrying the groceries back from the shops. It all counts.

CHAPTER SIX

Menu Plans

A new way of eating can be an exciting challenge as you discover new foods and ways of preparing them. If, however, you feel daunted by the prospect of making radical changes introduce new ideas gradually. These plans are intended to be guidelines for a hormone balancing approach to eating. Adapt them to suit your particular tastes and cooking style. But I would suggest you make one deal with yourself. If a food is unfamiliar, don't just dismiss it but make a point of using it in a few possible ways, and take the time to find new recipes or adapt old ones. This way you will widen your culinary horizons and give your diet a broader nutritional base.

There are two meal plans to experiment with. The second one is wheat-free since so many hormone balance problems, in particular premenstrual discomfort, are helped by avoiding this grain.

For snacks aim to stick to the healthier options such as fruit, fresh nuts and seeds, dried fruit or yoghurt. If you need something more satisfying have a cup of home-made soup (you can keep some portions in the freezer), or have something on a wholegrain cracker. Spreads could include guacamole, hummus, fish paté or nut butters, or you could have some prawns and coleslaw, chopped egg and cucumber or soya baked beans with crackers. Alternatively you can always keep some leftovers from your main meal options to snack on. The idea is to avoid reaching for the sweet snacks, or the packets of crisps.

For drinks stick to herb teas, coffee substitutes, vegetable juices, diluted fresh juices and herbal cocktails. Of course don't forget about water! Aim to keep alcohol to a minimum, and perhaps treat yourself a couple of times a week but no more.

Meal Plan One

Day	Breakfast	Lunch
1	Dried prunes and apricots soaked with linseeds topped with sheep's yoghurt.	Buckwheat kasha salad with goat's cheese.
2	Tofu and berry whiz.	Whole-wheat toast sandwich filled with hummus, finely sliced green pepper, red onion rings and crispy lettuce.
3	Porridge made with soya milk topped with ground linseeds and sunflower seeds.	Black bean and garlic soup with oatcakes.
4	Scrambled eggs with finely chopped onions, garlic and mushrooms (use 1 egg and 2 egg whites if keeping fat levels down).	Chilli-spiced soya beans with a green salad and quinoa.
5	Mashed banana on multi grain ryvita (with linseeds). Sprinkled with cinnamon.	Oatcakes spread with ricotta cheese topped with slices of beef tomatoes and basil leaves. Baked apple and live yoghurt.
6	Almond butter toast and a glass of soya milk.	Asparagus quiche made with wholemeal pastry. Served with tomato, tarragon and balsamic vinegar salad.
7	Rye crackers spread generously with mackerel pâté and cucumber slices.	Mixed bean salad with mandarin segments and yoghurt dressing.
8	Rye toast with soya baked beans in tomato sauce.	Cauliflower and broccoli cheese. Steam florets. In a large shallow dish spread with cottage cheese mixed with diced tomatoes and black olives. Grill.
9	Home made muesli made with soya flakes, rice flakes and roasted buckwheat groats, linseeds, pumpkin seeds and raisins. With yoghurt.	Red pepper stuffed with brown Basmati rice, chopped green olives, fennel and spring onions.
10	Papaya with ground linseeds mixed in soya yoghurt.	Wholemeal pitta stuffed with spinach leaves, avocado and beansprout salad topped with grilled halloumi cheese.

Meal Plan One

Evening	Day
Mixed mushrooms, sweetcorn and diced onions in a white sauce (made with soya milk) served with brown rice and broccoli spears.	1
Tuna and pasta bake (tuna, tinned tomatoes, capers, basil and wholemeal pasta) topped with grated soya cheese and grilled.	2
Grilled salmon steak (spread thinly with pesto) served with shredded savoy cabbage sprinkled with sesame seeds and mashed sweet potato.	3
Roast chicken with pickled red cabbage, roast sweet potatoes.	4
Seafood and tofu brown rice risotto. Served with watercress salad.	5
Vegetable curry on a bed of couscous and petit-pois. Garnish with chopped fresh coriander.	6
Fish pie made with an oat crumble topping served with carrots and kale.	7
Stir-fried vegetables (at least 3 colours) with marinated tofu served with kasha (cooked roasted buckwheat).	8
Tandoori chicken served with mange tout, orange rings with a ramekin of brown rice. Make the tandoori ckicken by dipping julienne chicken into curry spiced sheep's yoghurt and then grill.	9
Bulgar wheat, wild mushroom and leek risotto.	10

Meal Plan Two (wheat free)

Day	Breakfast	Lunch
1	In a glass layer soft fruit, yoghurt and soya flakes. Sprinkle linseeds on the last layer.	Mixed vegetable broth with barley.
2	Boiled egg and rice cakes.	Fennel and sprouted soya bean salad with cottage cheese, apricots and walnut halves.
3	Rolled oats and linseeds soaked in fruit juice. Have with goat's milk yoghurt.	Chargrilled vegetables with anchovies and capers.
4	Papaya squeezed with lime. Topped with live soya yoghurt.	Crustless leek and mushroom pie with grated beetroot in a lemon vinaigrette.
5	Grapefruit topped drizzled with honey and sprinkled with cinnamon and then grilled. Sesame ryvita spread with hazelnut butter.	Fanned tofu salad drizzled with tahini and ginger dressing. (Sliced marinated tofu, with sliced tomato, red onion rings and black olives).
6	Mackerel fillet coated in rolled oats and linseeds, fried in a little oil.	Brown rice and arugula leaf salad (Brown rice, watercress, sweet-corn, and pistachios).
7	Tropical tofu whiz made with tofu, mango and banana.	Baked potato and ratatouille.
8	Mini mushroom omelette.	Pepper crusted trout on endive leaves served with a warm lime and dill dressing.
9	Millet pops with soya milk, blackcurrants and seeds.	Bacon (lean), orange and avocado salad with parmesan flakes.
10	Fruit medley (choice of 3 types of chopped fruit) with coconut cream and linseeds.	Sardines on rye toast. Followed by an oven-warmed peach.

Meal Plan Two (wheat free)

Evening	Day
Lemon tarragon chicken served with new potatoes, runner beans and braised red cabbage.	1
Curried prawns in coconut milk served with brown rice.	2
Brown lentil casserole, spinach and roasted butternut squash.	3
Chilli chickpeas with Swiss chard leaves tossed in a pan of lightly fried garlic, onion. Sprinkled with sesame seeds.	4
Home-made salmon fishcakes (salmon, potato, finely sliced onion with parsley sauce. Serve with steamed green beans and ribbon carrots (sliced with a potato peeler).	5
Vegetable brochettes (grilled skewered button mushrooms, aubergines, onion wedges, courgettes and mozzarella coated with spicy tamari marinade made from garlic, cumin, olive oil, tamari). Served with wild rice and mixed leaf salad with lime and olive oil dressing.	6
Sweet and sour turkey with grilled pineapple rings and broccoli.	7
Buckwheat pasta with a tofu stir-fry (tofu, mini corn-cobs, mange tout, sliced spring onions, garlic and oregano). Serve with cherry tomato salad.	8
Shepherdess pie with julienne carrots and button Brussels sprouts (Shepherdess pie is vegetarian Shepherd's pie made with soya and kidney beans).	9
Vegetable and nut bake with mushroom sauce (sauce made with soya milk and wheat free flour).	10

Part Three

REDUCE

EXPOSURE

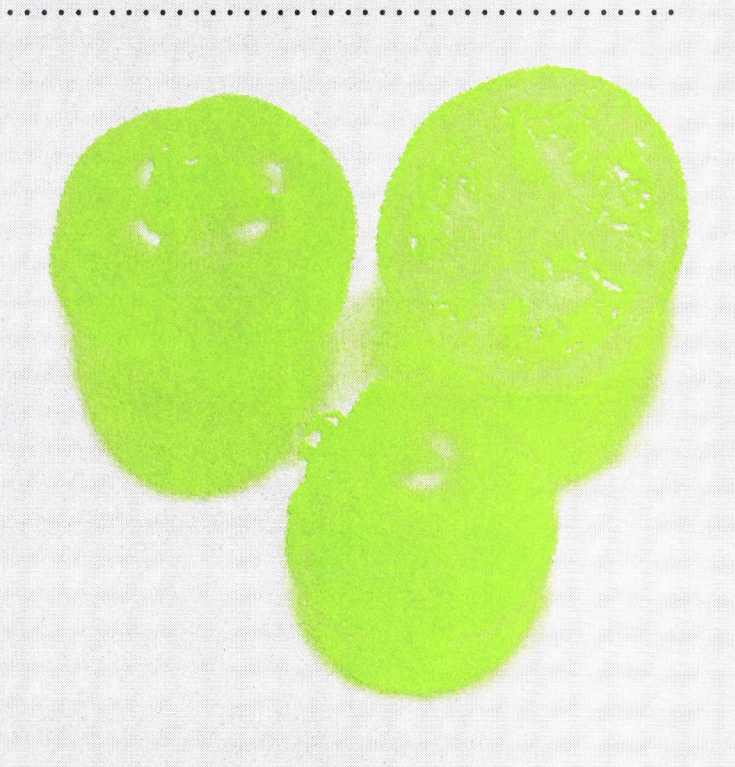

CHAPTER SEVEN

Cut Out Chemicals

Processing oestrogens out of your body, and balancing all your natural hormones (female, blood sugar, adrenal and thyroid hormones) is the foundation of hormone health, and the most important dietary steps have been covered in the 7-Point Plan. However, if you continue to be exposed to environmental oestrogens from your food, water and household chemicals it can remain an uphill battle for your body to achieve the desired balance.

The effect of these oestrogenic chemicals was discovered accidentally at Tufts University, USA. Two researchers, Ana Soto and Carlos Sonnenschein, were running experiments using plastic flasks. At one point it was noticed that the cells in the flasks were acting as if they were in the presence of oestrogens. After much sleuth work the researchers discovered that the manufacturers of the flasks had changed the make-up of them to include new compounds, which we now know to have an oestrogenic effect. It is now evident that a number of different plastics, agri-chemicals, petro-chemicals and other chemicals in our environment have similar effects. One aspect, of even more concern than the effects of the individual compounds, is the cumulative effect of these chemicals which are persistent, and build up in nature and in our bodies.

Go through the following checklist to cut back on your exposure to damaging xenoestrogens which may be contributing to your hormonal problems. Tackle each in turn, and seek out different products. It is no longer the case that only health food shops stock, for instance, detergent-free washing up liquids and washing powders. They are now generally stocked by supermarkets, though their labels are designed to appeal on the environment-friendly front, rather than the health-conscious one. Nevertheless, what is good for the environment is also good for your internal environment – or hormonal balance.

CHEMICALS IN OUR FOOD

- Eat organic food whenever you are able. The use of artificial pesticides and fertilisers is not allowed in organic food production and so this measure will significantly reduce your exposure to xenoestrogens. You can easily find organic vegetables, meat, dairy produce, bread and many other packaged products. If you are concerned about the cost of buying organic food, think for a moment about the foods which are least expensive and which can make up the bulk of any shopping basket. Root vegetables, fruit in season, grains and pulses are all relatively inexpensive and if you are planning to cut back on the more expensive items, in particular meat and packaged foods, you may find that with some careful planning, and a commitment to preparing more meals from fresh ingredients, that your weekly bill decreases rather than increases.
- Wash non-organic produce thoroughly in a bowl of water to which a tablespoon of vinegar has been added. This will help to strip away the waxy residue which retains the outer layer of sprays used. This does not, however, get rid of the chemicals in the fabric of the plant.
- Reduce fatty foods in your diet. Fats of all types, both animal and cooking oils, accumulate non-biodegradable chemicals. Cut visible fat off meat, reduce butter, margarine, cream, cheese and full- or semi-fat milk to a minimum. Eat

fresh nuts and seeds, and use olive oil, preferably all organic, for healthy sources of fats.
- Many cans, packets and drinks cartons have thin plastic linings inside them. These can leach oestrogenic compounds into the foods. Restrict foods in cans and cartons, such as canned fish or packaged fresh soups, to two or three times weekly as they are difficult to avoid totally. Buy items in glass bottles or jars whenever you have the option.

COOKING UTENSILS

- Use porcelain, glass or stainless steel cooking pans. Use ceramic storage containers, instead of plastic containers, especially for fatty foods. Do not heat your food in plastic containers – EVER.
- Use greaseproof paper instead of cling film food wrap. The more flexible a plastic is the more likely it is to leach xenoestrogens into food, especially into fatty foods such as meat, butter, cheese, biscuits, pastry, pies and so on. Shop bought foods in plastic are also a problem, especially fatty foods such as pies, chocolates, cheese and cold cuts. While it is difficult to avoid plastic bags coming into contact with food all the time, choose loose produce and paper bags whenever you can.

WATER QUALITY

- Use a water filter or, even better, distil your water, and buy mineral water in glass bottles.

HOUSEHOLD PRODUCTS

- Do not use pesticides in your garden, wood treatment in your house or pharmaceutical hair lice products. Herbal lice products are available, or use the wet combing method described in leaflets available at all chemists.
- Use natural detergents for washing dishes, clothes and also for general cleansing. Reputable companies will list the ingredients on the packaging.
- You can find unbleached alternatives for products such as tampons, coffee filters, tea bags, kitchen paper and lavatory paper in larger health food shops, as well as some supermarkets. Admittedly they will not be as attractively packaged and are more expensive, but you may feel it is worth using these options. Bleached products do not contribute directly to your oestrogenic load, but do so indirectly and significantly by their manufacture, which results in dioxin by-products. Dioxins are highly damaging oestrogenic compounds which are widespread environmental pollutants.

PERSONAL CARE

- You will find long lists of unpronounceable ingredients on everyday personal care and hygiene products. A significant number of these chemicals are substances you would not contemplate eating, and yet putting them on your skin is no wiser – we absorb a hefty amount through our skin. Aim to buy products with less, or no, chemicals in them. While these chemicals are unlikely to be oestrogenic, reducing your uptake of them will minimise your overall chemical load, and may be beneficial in the long run.
- Avoid using pharmaceutical hormone preparations such as the Pill and HRT. This topic is covered in detail in the next chapter.

CHAPTER EIGHT

Pills and Patches

In order to understand the merits of the natural approach to hormone balance, it is a good idea to review pharmaceutical hormones in the form of the contraceptive pill, HRT, SERMs and fertility treatments. We all have differing views about the appropriateness of using these little helpers. It is easy to understand the appeal of controlling our fertility, and extending youth – but there may be a price to pay.

An area that is deserving of attention is how pharmaceutical hormone use relates to nutritional status and overall health. If you are reading this book to find alternative options to drug use, this section will help to put the issues into perspective. Alternatively, if you are planning to use these drugs then this chapter can give you an idea of how to redress some of the balance.

The medicalisation of women's hormone problems has been driven to a large extent by the huge amount of money to be made by the pharmaceutical companies who sell these drugs. Potentially, all women between the ages of around 13 to 75, are a market for hormone drugs of one sort or another. The PR machinery which portrays the benefits of these is vast and has almost unlimited financial resources in selling their advantages to the medical profession and to the lay public.

Research into female hormone health has been largely spearheaded by men in the last century, and the truth is that managing female hormone health has been approached largely from the male perspective. Now that women are beginning to question this, the picture is altering somewhat, with more natural means being sought by a significant number of women.

THE CONTRACEPTIVE PILL

Since its launch in 1961, the Pill has, it seems, eliminated the last stumbling block to women's emancipation. Despite achieving the vote earlier in the century, women were still hampered in social and business advancement by their biological fate – that of fertility. The fact that the Pill offered women the opportunity to determine their reproductive life, made it an almost instant success, but it is only now, around 40 years later, that we are able to evaluate the statistical data and gauge the impact it may have had on the health of women.

The Pill is fairly unique amongst medications because it is usually given for social rather than for medical reasons, and in the UK it is now used by about 28 per cent of sexually active women.

A Tale of Two Pills

There are two types of Pill, the combined contraceptive and the progesterone only pill. Which one is prescribed depends on your medical history, though 98 per cent of women who take it use the combined pill.

Common side-effects of the Pill (listed in the drug formularies and information leaflets) include spotting and breakthrough bleeding, vaginal discharge, breast tenderness, weight changes, water retention, headaches, raised blood pressure, nausea, vomiting, depression, reduced sex drive, and, rarely, liver tumours. The oestrogen-based pills can also affect the impact of other drugs, meaning that caution must be taken about using other drugs alongside it. The oestrogens used in the Pill, mainly ethinyl oestradiol, are synthetic and stay in the body for many hours before they are excreted, unlike natural oestrogens which have a short life in the body. The oestrogen-based Pill can increase the risk of uterine fibroids, endometriosis, ovarian cysts

Combined Pill	Progestogen Pill
Effectiveness	
98–99 per cent	96-98 per cent
Hormones used	
Oestrogens and progestogens. Often phased to mimic the natural cycle	Progestogens only
Prescribed for	
Most women	When allergic to the Pill, or over 35, or heavy smokers, or if breast-feeding
Works by	
Mimicking pregnancy. Discouraging release of an egg	Mimicking pregnancy and making cervical mucus/uterus less receptive to sperm. Ovulation still happens in 60 per cent of cases but the eggs do not mature. Must be taken at the right time of day or may be ineffective.

and gall stones. The Pill does not increase hormone levels overall, but rather turns off the woman's own supply, while adding in a different type. It is the type of hormones which is the cause of doubt about long-term health associated with using the Pill. While long-term studies have shown that the risk of illnesses is not much greater for Pill users ten years after using the Pill, there is a slight increase in breast cancer risk. The group of women who are most likely to be affected by increased breast cancer risk are the most vulnerable group – women who take it in their teens when breast tissue is even more sensitive to its effects. The most serious health risk is related to thrombosis, which affects 15–30 in 100,000 users (compared to 5 in 100,000 non-users). The progestogen only Pills have irregular menstrual cycles, raised blood pressure, ovarian cysts and ectopic pregnancies as the main risk factors. Cautions are made regarding jaundice.

The Pill can affect the immune system and can lower the antigen-antibody response, which can increase the likelihood of hayfever, asthma and other allergies and infections such as cystitis. Urinary tract infections (cystitis) and yeast infections are often aggravated by using the Pill. See measures to help these in **Thrush and Cystitis** page 112.

A strong argument in favour of the Pill is that the risks, especially of fatalities, are considerably less than the risks attached to terminating unwanted pregnancies or even carrying pregnancies to full term, where the baby may also put a stress on the mother if not really wanted. These are difficult issues to resolve and are very personal ones, however strictly from the perspective of the health of the woman who is taking the Pill, it is helpful to have the nutritional information outlined in this chapter to help redress the balance. Mothers of young girls taking the Pill may want to discuss some of this information with them. A brand of Pill, Dianette, is frequently prescribed for women with acne, but the problem with this approach is that it does not seek to resolve the underlying causes, and the acne is likely to return when the Pill is stopped. The Pill is also prescribed to women to resolve severe PMS, and again this simply resolves the symptoms and does not look at the causes.

THE CONTRACEPTIVE PILL AFFECTS NUTRITIONAL STATUS

Most women are unaware that the contraceptive pill can have a profound effect on the way the body handles nutrients. This factor can be instrumental in different women's response to the medication.

The liver is one major organ to be affected, as the oestrogen hormones are metabolised by the liver. Caffeine can increase the time it takes for oral contraceptives to clear through the liver, and this may increase the likelihood of experiencing side-effects. The Pill can also lower the clearance rate of alcohol from the body, probably because of its effect on the enzyme systems of the liver.

If you are taking oral contraceptives, a good diet becomes doubly important. Oestrogens can encourage water retention, meaning that it is best to reduce salt to keep water retention under control. High levels of refined sugar, carbohydrates and alcohol can contribute to blood sugar problems, as well as contributing indirectly to raised blood cholesterol, both of which can be worsened by the Pill.

Pill use can also reduce levels of B vitamins, including folic acid. It is very important to supplement folic acid at levels of 400–800 mcg daily if you are coming off the Pill because you want to conceive, since low folic acid levels have been linked to neural tube defects in developing babies. Continue to take this level for at least the three months after coming off the Pill and prior to conception. After this, drop back to a maintenance dose of 400 mcg, and keep this up until you conceive and for at least the first trimester of the pregnancy. It is also a good idea to take a 50–100 mg B-complex supplement if you have recently been on the Pill, to make up for any losses. This is particularly important for vegetarians or vegans, who have a higher risk of vitamin B12 deficiency, since taking the Pill makes the risk of deficiency more acute. Food sources of the B-vitamins are wholegrains, brewer's yeast, liver, green leafy vegetables, wheatgerm, figs, dates, eggs, yoghurt, apricots, avocados, molasses and oily fish.

Likewise zinc and manganese levels are depleted by the Pill. Zinc is critical for the developing foetus, and so supplementing with around 25 mg daily is advised if you have been on the Pill for a while. Food sources of zinc are meat, all seeds, nuts, wholegrains, brewer's yeast, wheatgerm, egg yolks, cauliflower, berries, lettuce and tuna. Manganese can be taken at levels between 5–100 mg daily. Manganese is poorly absorbed and some people may need more than others. Food sources of manganese are nuts, green leafy vegetables, peas, beetroot, egg yolks and wholegrains.

Vitamin C, too, is depleted by the Pill, as are the bioflavanoids which make vitamin C more effective and which are found naturally alongside vitamin C in foods. This is possibly because the Pill causes vitamin C to be broken down more quickly in the body. However, supplemented vitamin C should only be taken at the level of around 1000mg daily by those currently on the Pill. Some research has shown that vitamin C reacts with the synthetic oestrogen in the Pill, and has the effect of turning a low-dose Pill into a high-dose Pill, and this may increase susceptibility to thrombosis. If you are taking a higher level of vitamin C than this, it is necessary to reduce the dose slowly over a period of around 14 days. If it is decreased too quickly, there is a chance of breakthrough bleeding or even pregnancy resulting, as it is similar to moving from a high-dose Pill to a low-dose Pill. Vitamin C has no detrimental effect on naturally produced oestrogens or on oestrogen-related ailments if you are not on the Pill. The converse is true, however, if you are, and vitamin C can probably help to reduce the risk of many diseases, including hormone-related cancers. Vitamin C rich foods include all fruits, especially citrus, kiwis, strawberries, cantaloupes, most vegetables, especially sweet potatoes, potatoes, green leafy vegetables (i.e. cabbage), cauliflowers and turnips.

There is some suggestion that supplemented vitamin K may be a risk with the Pill. This is because the Pill increases the risk of blood clotting, and vitamin K is the vitamin which is responsible for helping the clotting process. However vitamin K is rarely put into vitamin supplements and is not widely available as a separate supplement. It is becoming popular in preparations designed to avoid osteoporosis, but those taking such preparations are usually women beyond the age of Pill use. Food sources of vitamin K include cauliflowers, green leafy vegetables, yoghurt, alfalfa, egg yolks, safflower oil, kelp, milk.

The Pill raises levels of vitamin A, copper and iron in the blood. Vitamin A stores in the liver are channelled into the blood, meaning that liver stores can be depleted while blood levels are raised. Some authorities have suggested that this means that supplemented vitamin A in excess of that found in a typical multivitamin supplement (7,500 ius) is inadvisable. This would mean taking care with antioxidant supplements and cod liver oil, both of which contain vitamin A. However, there is dissent about this fact, and it does not seem likely that this is a great problem. If you want to be cautious though you may want to restrict yourself to taking beta-carotene which converts into vitamin A, but is non-toxic as it is water soluble. Zinc is needed to make this conversion, and so supplementing 15,000–25,000 ius (international units) of beta-carotene would need 5–15 mg of zinc alongside it. Food sources of vitamin A are liver, cod-liver oil, egg yolks, full fat dairy produce, herrings, mackerel and other oily fish.

Copper levels are raised by accelerating the liver's production of a copper binding protein. Abnormally elevated copper in turn interferes with zinc and manganese absorption. Iron levels are often raised because of decreased blood loss with lighter menstruation while on the Pill. Avoid using copper and iron cooking utensils, and make sure that you use stainless steel or ceramic options.

It may be inadvisable to take herbs which have an oestrogenic effect while on the Pill. Some of these are described in **Herbs for Harmony** on page 85. Feverfew is also suspect as it was once used to bring on suppressed menstruation. In fact, herbs are always best taken on the advice of a qualified herbalist, especially if you are taking any medication, as there can be interactions with many different types of drug, not just the Pill.

No significant information is available about interactions between progestogens and nutrients, and it appears that oestrogens have a more profound effect on the body's nutritional status. This means that taking HRT will have a similar nutritional effect to that just described for the Pill.

STOPPING THE PILL

If you have decided to stop taking the Pill, you should find that your periods return to their pre-Pill pattern without too much trouble. Of course, this may mean a return to your pre-Pill PMS, in which case turn to the chapter **Moontime Madness** on page 117.

You should always allow at least three months, and preferably six, before attempting to conceive, and you will need to use barrier, or timing, methods of contraception during this time (see **Fertility**, page 129).

In around two per cent of women, menstruation is suppressed and can take as long as six months to resume. If it goes on for this long, it is best to check with your doctor. Of the women who do not resume menstruation post-Pill, 40 per cent will notice a clear or milky discharge from the nipple(s). This is called galactorrhoea and usually stops when menstruation finally returns to normal.

PROGESTOGENS – NOT PROGESTERONE BY ANOTHER NAME

In the early days of oestrogen and progesterone research, the two hormones were isolated from the ovaries of animals, and literally thousands of animals would be sacrificed to produce a few milligrams of usable hormone. The only other source of sex hormones was from frozen placentas. By the 1940s scientists made a breakthrough and learnt to synthesize progesterone from plant roots, at a viable cost. In the 1950s the first artificial progestogen was developed which could be administered orally without being destroyed by the digestive tract.

Unlike oestrogens, where there are several different types (the term oestrogen really refers to a class of hormones), there is only one progesterone. Progesterone is a relatively benign hormone which is produced at a time in our cycles when we are likely to be nurturing new life – which means that it has to be pretty safe, as long it is used appropriately. But the downside of any natural hormone is that it cannot be patented, and there is no real money to be made out of natural substances when compared to patented formulas. For this reason research during the 1950s concentrated on producing a number of artificial progesterones – called progestogens in the UK and progestins in the US. These substances are patentable, so they are big business.

The Pill and HRT both use artificial progestogens. And yet for a hormone that is meant to be produced by the body at times of pregnancy, one of the main contra-indications of some progestogens is that they are not to be used when planning a pregnancy, as they can be responsible for early miscarriages or birth defects. So much for the benign nature of these artificial hormones. Artificial progestogens have also been linked to cardiovascular problems, cervical erosion, decreased glucose tolerance, acne and depression, plus they do not build new bone, which progesterone does. The only reason that progestogens are put in the Pill and HRT at all is because they moderate the damaging effects of the oestrogens, not because they have health benefits in their own right.

HRT – HORMONE REPLACEMENT THERAPY

Along with the Pill, HRT appears to offer women the Golden Chalice. Eternal youth has been sought for centuries, and seemingly by replacing hormones which are the wellspring of our younger years, we can continue to enjoy their benefits into later years. The menopause does not sound very appealing if you listen to the advertising pushed out by the drug companies: hot flushes, dry vagina, crumbling bones and a heart-disease risk which mirrors that of men. No wonder women are tempted to consider HRT. And with little time to discuss the options, the time-pressured GP does not have the resources to discuss preventive options. If a man with a possible cardiovascular risk goes into the doctor's surgery, it will often be suggested that he cuts back on salt, reduces his dependency on saturated fats, eats oats, exercises more and stops smoking – all known modulators of heart disease risk. But if a woman of a certain age consults her doctor she will commonly be offered HRT with the accompanying advice that it reduces the risk of heart disease – with little, or no, dietary or lifestyle counselling. Doctors discuss HRT with 89 per cent of women aged between 35–54, and yet only 17 per cent of women try it.

HRT does not suit all women and only one in ten continues with it for more than a year, because of adverse side effects. There is great concern about the clear evidence which shows that HRT increases the chance of hormone-related cancers, especially breast cancer. The reason that this happens seems to be quite straightforward – by taking HRT a woman is exposing herself to a greater amount of oestrogen, and this leads to an escalation of tissue growth in sensitive organs such as the breast. The type of oestrogen used in the Pill and in HRT, ethinyl oestradiol, is not the same hormone that we produce in our bodies, making it suspicious in terms of its long-term effects on whole body health. Contra-indications and cautions for HRT list: migraines, a history of thrombosis, liver disease, a family history of breast cancer, fibroids, endometriosis. Given how common problems such as fibroids, endometriosis and having family members with breast cancer is, it is no surprise that HRT is deemed to not suit a great number of women. If you are tempted to use HRT then it would seem that patches are preferable to pills. This is because 17ß-oestradiol, the hormone we produce in our bodies is well absorbed through the skin, and this is the hormone used. The pills use conjugated oestrogens which have to be turned into 17ß-oestradiol in the liver.

SERMs

SERMs stands for Selective oEstrogen Receptor Modulators, and these are the latest class of hormone drugs which have caused great excitement amongst the medical community. As the name implies SERMs affect the impact that oestrogens can have on the oestrogen receptor sites on cells of sensitive tissues. The effects of SERMs is sometimes not very easy to explain and may, for instance, have an oestrogen dampening effect on some body tissues, while having an oestrogen enhancing effect on others.

The best known SERM is Tamoxifen, which is used as a hormone treatment for breast cancer in 80 per cent of women diagnosed with the disease. This is a drug which has only been in use for about 15 years and so it is still being evaluated intensively. The early results seem to show that it is having some positive effects, with a 15 per cent drop in breast cancer mortality rates in the last few years which may be attributable to Tamoxifen. On the other hand, there are potential side effects that may discourage some women from using it, especially if, as is now suggested, Tamoxifen is used preventatively in women who have not yet had breast cancer. These side effects may also increase in severity with longer-term use – it is unlikely that any women have taken it for longer than seven to ten years, so at this stage we do not really know. Side effects include being tipped into an early menopause, eye sight disruption (reversible), an increase in endometrial cancers and even a possibility of liver cancer. As with any drug, it is a case of weighing up the benefits, which may be significant, against the possible longer-term problems.

Other SERMs are now coming onto the market, such as Raloxifen/Evista. These drugs are being recommended as an alternative option for women who do not want to take, or cannot take, HRT, though they do not influence hot flushes. It is claimed that such drugs increase bone density and reduce the risk of fractures without increasing the risk of breast cancer (which is associated with HRT). These claims were criticised in Drug and Therapeutics Bulletin (published by *Which?*) as being not fully substantiated, further trials being needed. In any event, as with any new drug, caution must be employed by anyone considering taking something for which long-term evidence is not available.

The viewpoint of therapists working with natural medicine is that there are a number of foods which offer oestrogen-modulating effects and can be viewed as natural SERMs. These foods are mainly soya, legumes and grains. If women incorporate these into their diet on a regular basis, while at the same time reducing mineral-leaching foods, they can positively influence bone mineral density as well as reduce the risk of cardiovascular disease and breast cancer and help allay menopausal problems such as hot flushes.

FERTILITY TREATMENT

The whole question of hormone therapy is an emotive one, and none more so than fertility treatment. It is understandable that couples who are infertile, and who desperately want to start a family, are tempted by the possibility of fertility treatment.

Fertility drugs work by a variety of methods. Some will trigger an increase in FSH (follicle stimulating hormone) and LH (luteinising hormone). This can encourage ovulation to take place. Other drugs actually mimic the hormones FSH or hCG (human chorionic gonadotrophic hormone), with the same results. Another option is IVF (in vitro fertilisation) where hormones are used to stimulate the production of eggs which are fertilised outside the body and then re-implanted. Alternatively, the eggs may come from a donor. In either case hormones are used on the woman carrying the baby to maintain the pregnancy in the early stages.

The immediate and obvious downside of these hormone drug treatments is that there are side effects. These can include, depending on the drugs used, hot flushes, nausea, headaches and, sometimes, ovarian cysts. Additionally, any drug fertility treatment which stimulates ovulation increases blood copper levels. This can force down zinc levels, and low zinc levels are linked to reproductive problems. There is also a possibility that fertility drugs raise the risk of ovarian cancer later in life due to increased activity in the ovaries.

The unquantifiable, and rather scarier effect, which has been suggested as a possibility, is that the hormones used may affect the next generation. A female foetus will have her full complement of several million eggs in place in her ovaries by the 12th week of gestation. This means that there is a real possibility that hormones used at that time will affect the health of the baby girl's eggs. This is totally unproven, and there is a risk that mentioning it may be viewed as scaremongering, but I believe that it is necessary to know of this possibility as these treatments are still relatively new and we do not understand what their full implications may be down the generations. As it is we definitely know that babies produced by IVF have double the chance of being born with congenital defects.

There is work being done by a dedicated organisation, Foresight, which concerns itself with pre-conceptual care. Foresight claims that, as long as there is no structural defect such as blocked fallopian tubes, 80 per cent of infertility cases can be resolved by attention to a number of factors. These factors include:

- A wholefood diet to get the best sources of nutrients to start a new life.
- Making up nutrient deficiencies. Tests are run to work out which vitamins or minerals the individual is maybe lacking. A balance of these nutrients is needed for optimising a healthy pregnancy.
- Dealing with genito-urinary infections, such as chlamydia, to reduce the chance of early miscarriage.
- Eliminating toxic heavy metals such as lead (from water pipes) and cadmium (from cigarette smoke) which can interfere with the healthy development of a baby.
- Both partners are treated.

Foresight also claim that many couples who have tried IVF unsuccessfully have succeeded in conceiving after following their programme. Given the mental, financial and possibly chemical price that artificial hormone treatment may have, it probably makes sense to follow such a programme for at least a year to see if it yields results, before embarking on hormone treatments for infertility.

Part Four

NATURAL HORMONES

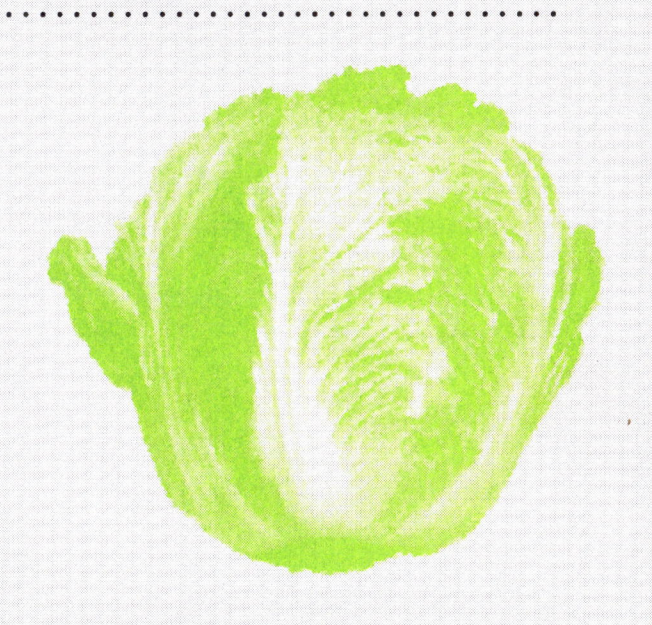

CHAPTER NINE

Phytohealth

For many millennia we have been evolving in harmony with nature, and our bodies have adapted to use the benefits which plants can offer us. One of the great research discoveries of recent years is that plants are sources of compounds which are capable of moderating our own hormones. Many of these plants have been used by herbalists throughout history to manipulate hormones – for contraception, fertility or even to induce abortions.

These compounds have been dubbed phytohormones. Phyto just means plants, and plants can be sources of both phytoestrogens and phyto-progesterones. In the last decade there has been particular interest in phytoestrogens, which have the ability to balance our hormones.

Oestrogens, produced in the body, or from outside sources, circulate in the blood and then attach to cells in sensitive organs, such as breasts, the uterus and the cervix. They attach to the cells at specific areas called receptor sites, which are a little like docking terminals. The hormones lock onto these terminals to carry out their business.

If the hormones which lock onto these sites are the strong or damaging oestrogens, they send out magnified messages to the cells to behave in a particular way. They can influence the tissues to speed up growth and to become more swollen. This can result in swollen breasts, lumps, fibroids and even female hormone dependent cancers such as breast, ovarian and endometrial cancers.

Phytoestrogens are remarkable because they can also lock

onto these receptor sites and have an effect on them. However, they are much gentler hormone sources than either our naturally produced body oestrogens, or the xenoestrogens to which we are exposed from the environment. When they lock onto the receptor sites they have an effect, but they are between 100–1000 times weaker than other sources of oestrogens. Not only is their effect weaker, but they also block the receptor sites, which means that stronger oestrogens which are circulating are not able then to lock onto the receptors. In this way they protect us against the negative effects of damaging oestrogens.

These phytoestrogens also have another remarkable health benefit. When our natural oestrogen levels diminish, as we approach the menopause or are beyond it, phytoestrogens can have a hormone replacement effect. There is a strong body of research showing that phytoestrogens from foods, and herbs, have a positive effect on the early effects of the menopause, such as hot flushes and vaginal dryness, as well as on the longer-term potential problems such as cardiovascular disease, osteoporosis and breast cancer (see **Managing Your Menopause**, page 151).

SOURCES OF PHYTOESTROGENS

There are around 300 known sources of phytoestrogens. Including a wide variety of plant foods in your diet is the best way forward in helping to balance out hormones. Foods which have the greatest amounts include:

Soya foods: including soya beans, soya flour, soya flakes, soya mince, soya yoghurt, soya milk, tofu, tempeh and miso
Whole grains: such as brown rice, wholewheat, barley, rye, millet, corn and buckwheat
Legumes: for instance, chickpeas, peas, peanuts, lentils, lima beans, mung beans and pinto beans

Seeds and nuts: such as sunflower seeds, sesame seeds, linseeds (flax seeds) and almonds

Vegetables and fruits: fennel, celery, parsley, green beans, alfalfa sprouts, any sprouted beans, grains and seeds, seaweed, spinach, mushrooms, rhubarb, apples, grapes and citrus fruit

The most potent sources of phytoestrogens from foods are soya products, linseeds, wholewheat, rye and chickpeas. The phytoestrogens in soya foods, called isoflavones, have been the subject of intense study in recent years, particularly in respect of their hormone-moderating effects which influence menopausal symptoms, osteoporosis, heart disease and breast cancer.

Interest was initiated when the vast differences in the incidence of some diseases which exist between societies on different diets suggested that eating soya foods might have a protective effect against these health problems. For instance in Japan, an industrialised county, the incidence of breast cancer is a quarter of that in the UK and US, and they have no word in their language for hot flushes. They have similarly impressive statistics for other hormone-dependent diseases such as prostate cancer. It has been of great interest that Eastern societies, such as the Japanese and the Chinese, have completely different hormone health profiles which cannot be explained by genetics – the differences rapidly dissolved when women from these other cultures moved to Western countries and adopted the local diet. Equally, when Western women moved to an Eastern country and adopted the local diet their health risks changed to those of the local population.

Subsequent research has suggested that the isoflavone phytoestrogens in soya are very important in influencing the situation. It has been found that a level of 50 mg of isoflavones has a significant effect on preventing the incidence of hormonal problems. Some people find that eating large amounts of soya does not agree with them if they introduce it too quickly. It is best to restrict soya foods to five days a week, and to introduce them slowly into your regime over a period of two or three months.

Phytoestrogen/isoflavone levels of soya foods

Soya flakes	1/2 cup	130 mg
Soya flour	1/2 cup	85 mg
TVP (soya mince)	1/2 cup	70 mg
Soya beans, cooked	100 gms	35 mg
Soya beans, sprouted	100 gms	35 mg
Tempeh	1/2 cup	35 mg
Tofu (full fat)	100 mg	30 mg
Tofu (low fat)	100 mg	20 mg
Soya yoghurt	100 gms	15 mg
Soya milk (full fat)	1 cup	10 mg
Soya milk (low fat)	1 cup	5 mg
Miso	1 tbsp	5 mg
Soya cheese	100 mg	3 mg

*All cup measurements use standard kitchen measuring cups

One potential problem is that soya is one of the main crops to have been used extensively in the new science of genetic modification (GM). Nobody yet knows what the likely effects of GM engineering is on the benefits of soya isoflavones. Until we know more about this massive experiment on human health I would suggest that you buy organic soya products, as they are free of GM soya.

Before embarking on regimes of taking supplemented herbs, or even natural hormones, it is wise to start with increasing levels of soya foods and other phytoestrogen-rich foods in your diet. Other ways of incorporating these foods into your diet are covered in point 4 of the 7-Point Plan.

CHAPTER TEN

Herbs for Harmony

Herbs have a long history of use in helping to relieve female hormone problems, both in the European and the Eastern herbal traditions. We now have the benefit of many years of experience of their use, and clinical trials have also been conducted for many herbs.

Herbs can be extremely powerful, which makes them effective for dealing with PMS and menopausal symptoms, however they should never be taken during pregnancy or while breastfeeding. You should also not take herbs alongside medication of any sort, and especially not alongside the Pill or HRT, as they can interact. The only exception to this is if they have been prescribed by a qualified herbalist.

Many women find tremendous relief from their hormonal ailments with the use of some of the herbs described below. Good herbal companies will also supply herbal supplements offering a mixture of synergistic herbs, and sometimes nutrients which are designed to work together for maximum therapeutic effect.

Dong Quai

It is the tap-root of dong quai that is used as a remedy. Also known as 'angelica', dong quai is an incredibly useful herb as it alleviates almost all symptoms which relate to problems of the female reproductive system. It is especially effective at reducing hot flushes, as well as other menopausal symptoms, and is also an effective remedy for PMS and irregular and painful periods. In the Far East it is known as the female adaptogen, meaning that it adapts and regulates female hormone imbalances. It is the medicinal herb most commonly used by Asian women. Side effects from using this herb are rare, but it has been known, when taken in high doses, to cause bloating, and it may affect the timing of the menstrual cycle.

How to use it:

For PMS take dong quai from day 14 of your cycle (time of ovulation) until the start of your period.

For painful periods take dong quai from day 14 of your cycle until the end of your period.

For the menopause dong quai can be used at any time

Dose: 2–6 grams of dried root equivalent three times a day.

Black Cohosh

Black cohosh has a phytoestrogen effect and is useful for oestrogen dominance problems (possibly caused by environmental oestrogens), even when there is low oestrogen, such as in the menopause. This is why, although black cohosh can help to reduce fibroids and relieve premenstrual syndrome, as well as painful periods and breast tenderness, it is particularly useful for the transition through the menopause. It was originally used by American Indians to help minimise menopausal symptoms and, even today, it is the most commonly used herb for the menopause. Research studies have shown that it is as effective as HRT and has far fewer side effects.

Black cohosh is an exceptionally powerful herb, and it is precisely because of its effectiveness that it should be used with care. In excess, black cohosh can result in problems with balance, vision and mood.

Dose: 0.2–1 gram of dried rhizome equivalent three times a day.

Liquorice Root

Liquorice root is used to encourage female hormone balance by competing with oestrogen and so it is useful in cases of oestrogen dominance. The great benefit of liquorice is that it also raises progesterone levels by stopping progesterone from being broken down. This leaves more of it available to the cells of the body. Liquorice is also useful for reducing premenstrual bloating.

Unfortunately liquorice sweets are no good, but you can get liquorice root from health food shops. It looks just like a twig but it has a strong sweet liquorice flavour. As tasty as it may be, any form of liquorice root should not be taken in excessive amounts and must not be used if you have a history of high blood pressure, other cardiovascular problems or kidney problems. The side effects of taking liquorice are that it increases the loss of potassium from the body and increases the retention of sodium, which means it can result in water retention and bloating. It may be advisable to boost your intake of potassium-rich foods (all fruits and vegetables) and avoid salt while using liquorice.

How to use it: Should be taken around ovulation, approximately day 14 of your cycle until your period starts.

Dose: 1–4 grams of dried fresh herb equivalent three times per day.

Chasteberry

Chasteberries grow on a native Mediterranean shrub, which has blue or white flowers. This shrub is also known as *vitex agnus castus*, which is why the name *agnus castus* is also used for chasteberry remedies.

As the name implies, chasteberry, if given in high enough doses, could be described as an herbal chastity belt! The berries' powerful ability to affect female hormones is why, traditionally, chasteberry remedies were given to young women to dampen down their sex drive! We get a good idea why it is also referred to as monk's pepper! However these, perhaps undesirable, effects are not evident in smaller doses. Using the correct doses for an individual, chasteberry mimics the action of the corpus luteum, which produces progesterone. This is why, in the case of oestrogen dominance, it can correct the balance of oestrogen to progesterone.

While black cohosh is the most popular herbal remedy for the menopause, chasteberry is the most commonly used herbal remedy for the relief of PMS. Because it is so effective, it is best taken on the advice of a health practitioner who can monitor the changes in your hormone levels.

Dose: 1 gram dried fruit equivalent three times a day.

Motherwort

Motherwort is also known as lion's ear. Little is known about motherwort in comparison to the other herbs which are commonly used to help correct hormone imbalances. It is assumed to have oestrogenic activity and is used for disturbed menstrual cycles. Its greatest use is, perhaps, for painful periods that are accompanied with mood fluctuations and tension.

Dose: 1–4 grams of dried herb equivalent three times a day.

Alfalfa

Alfalfa is a herb which is packed full of nutrients and has a phyto-oestrogen effect, which is why it is used to balance hormones, in particular where there is oestrogen dominance. It is a rich plant indeed! The nutrients it contains include the range of B vitamins, vitamins C and E, carotenoids, which can be converted to vitamin A, plus the minerals calcium, potassium and iron. It also contains protein. Although alfalfa can be taken in powdered form, sprouting alfalfa seeds have hundreds of times the nutrient content. Alfalfa sprouts make a good change from cress in sandwiches and can be added to give salads a refreshing difference.

Dose: 3–10 grams of dried herb equivalent three times a day.

Red Clover

Red clover has been used for hundreds of years for coughs and for the clearing of mucus from the lungs. Now, however, in the era of hormone problems, it is being used for its phytoestrogen activity to help imbalanced sex hormones and for menopause symptoms.

Dose: 3–6 grams of dried flower equivalent three times per day.

Sage

This herb is a prime remedy for night sweats and hot flushes which can accompany the menopause. It may be effective because it directly decreases production of sweat. It combines well with motherwort for treating these problems. It also has a regulatory effect on menstruation and is helpful for irregular periods, painful periods and heavy bleeding. Sage is also a brain and nerve tonic, and is helpful for promoting calmness and clarity of mind – which can be a boon if you feel thrown off course by your hormones. As well as using both purple and green sage as culinary herbs, you can make a tea by steeping the dried herb in boiling water for five minutes.

Dose: 1–4 grams dried herb equivalent three times daily.

Sarsaparilla

This tongue twister has a progesterone-like effect which can help in cases of progesterone deficiency. It is useful for PMS, low libido and vaginal itching. Because it also has a testosterone effect it is used to help to build up muscle, and may be not advised for women with PCOS (polycystic ovary syndrome). Sarsaparilla is usually combined in preparations with other herbs, particularly black cohosh.

Dose: 1-4 grams dried root equivalent three times daily.

CHAPTER ELEVEN

Natural Hormones

Information about synthetic hormones is available from your doctor, as is information about natural hormones, though the latter have not been as widely marketed. However, because natural hormones are identical in structure to the hormones we produce in our bodies, they are more sympathetic to our physiology and have a more useful effect with fewer downsides.

NATURAL PROGESTERONE

Most of the hormonal problems discussed in this book have related to an excess of oestrogens being manufactured naturally by the body, or from xenoestrogens from chemicals in our food, water, plastics and household products. One of the roles of progesterone is to oppose, or moderate, oestrogens, thus when levels of progesterone are low this means that oestrogens can have a greater impact. By balancing out the effects of oestrogens, progesterone can promote hormonal health and reduce a number of adverse symptoms, including some of the more debilitating ones such as fibroids and endometriosis.

HOW THE BODY USES PROGESTERONE

The effects of progesterone are far-reaching:

- It balances out oestrogen levels, which makes it of paramount importance in women with oestrogen dominance.
- It is used as the parent hormone to make other hormones

when needed. These include the three main oestrogens, as well as testosterone, cortisol (a stress hormone) and aldosterone (which influences water balance), plus other steroid hormones.
- It increases the effectiveness of thyroid hormones so that, if you are using thyroid medication alongside progesterone, you may need to consult your doctor about lowering the thyroxine.
- It turns up the body's thermostat, which makes it easier to burn fat.
- It improves the ability of the cells to maintain proper oxygen levels, which is important for metabolism and may help to prevent cancer.
- It may be protective against female hormone problems, including fibrocystic breasts, endometriosis, fibroids, polycystic ovaries, breast cancer, endometrial cancer.

Natural progesterone as a product is, in one sense, not natural at all. It is manufactured in a laboratory and is made from a substance called diosgenin which is extracted from yams or soya. The resulting manufactured progesterone is identical to the naturally produced hormone made in our bodies – hence the name. We, however, are unable to convert diosgenin into progesterone in our bodies when we take in yam. Products which are derived from yams will have very limited hormonal effects. As a herb, yam has traditionally been used as an antispasmodic and anti-inflammatory remedy, not for hormonal balance.

HOW TO USE NATURAL PROGESTERONE

Natural progesterone is available as a cream which you rub on in small amounts. The exact amount depends on what you are using it for, and it is best to seek the advice of your doctor. It is best to use the cream on different areas of the body in rotation. If you follow the manufacturers' recommended dose the creams deliver a 'physiological' dose of around 15–20 mg of hormone daily – about the same amount that your body produces in a day. Artificial progestogens have much more hard-hitting dosages. The cream is absorbed into the fatty layer just under the skin, and from there it is taken up by the blood and directed to where it is needed. Cells which are sensitive to it have progesterone receptor sites which allow them to respond to the hormone.

Some typical programmes are as follows below. Day 1 of the cycle is the first day of your period. Day 14 is deemed to be the middle of your cycle when most women ovulate. Day 28 is the last day of your cycle. If you have a different cycle pattern to this you will need to adjust the schedule accordingly, but always take Days 1–14 as the same, shortening or lengthening the second part of your cycle as appropriate. Do not follow these programmes slavishly as they are given as a guide only, and check with your doctor to see if they are suitable for your needs.

Probably the best way of reminding yourself to use the cream is to use it when you brush your teeth morning and evening. It can be used like a cosmetic cream on any area, but is most effective on areas where it is readily absorbed, such as on the face, neck, breasts, abdomen, inner arm or inner thigh. Start with the recommended dose of 15–20 mg (using the scoop provided with the cream) and then adjust the dose up or down according to your need. This is not difficult to assess once you become accustomed to using the cream and are aware of how it affects you. You can discuss this with your prescribing doctor. If you have any adverse symptoms stop using the cream until you talk to your doctor.

Premenstrual symptoms

The progesterone cream is used in a way that simulates the natural cycle, with none used for the first half of the cycle, followed by steadily increasing levels for the last half:

DAY 1 to DAY 13	Do not use the cream
DAY 14 to DAY 17	Use 1/8 tsp twice daily
DAY 18 to DAY 22	Use 1/4 tsp twice daily
DAY 23 to DAY 28	Use 1/2 tsp twice daily

Menopausal symptoms and post-menopausal care

Needs at the peri-menopausal time vary from woman to woman, and you may need to adjust your use accordingly. Use the schedule below as a rough guide only. If you are post-menopausal (you have stopped menstruating) then base your dates on the calendar month for ease.

DAY 1 to DAY 6	Do not use the cream
DAY 7 to DAY 20	Use 1/4 tsp twice daily
DAY 21 to DAY 28	Use 1/2 tsp twice daily

Persistent menopausal symptoms

If you find that using natural progesterone according to the schedule above does not relieve persistent vaginal dryness, you can see if applying the natural progesterone vaginally improves it, possibly alongside oestriol cream also applied to the vaginal area (see **Natural Oestrogen** on page 97).

If persistent hot flushes remain a problem, use a quarter teaspoon every 15 minutes for one hour following the hot flush (a total of four times).

Another option is to use natural progesterone oil, which can be more effective for persistent menopausal symptoms. Place 2–5 drops of the oil under your tongue, and if necessary repeat every 15 minutes for one hour after the hot flush (a total of four doses).

Bone re-mineralisation

The first step to take is to have a bone density scan to understand exactly what condition your bones are in. You can have follow-up scans each year thereafter to monitor the extent to which they are improving with treatment. Follow the treatment plan below, however, if you have severe osteoporosis, or if you have previously suffered any fractures, then double the dose by increasing the dosage slowly. See **Reversing Osteoporosis** on page 159.

DAY 1 to DAY 6	Do not use the cream
DAY 7 to DAY 28	Use 1/8–1/4 tsp twice daily

Cautionary Tales

Natural progesterone is not the one answer to every woman's hormone problems, even though it can sometimes seem as if it is being portrayed in this way. It is certainly of enormous benefit in a number of cases, but it is important not to invest it with powers beyond its capabilities. There is debate amongst advocates of natural medicine about where natural progesterone fits into the spectrum. My own experience is that, if it is used wisely, natural progesterone is of immense benefit. However, it is not a panacea, and it is unwise to use it at the expense of resolving nutritional and lifestyle issues first of all.

There are other cautions. If you are pre-menopausal, remember that progesterone is the hormone which is intended to promote pregnancy and it is entirely possible that you will find that you are more fertile as a result of using the cream. If you do not wish to get pregnant see the section on natural family planning in **Fertility** page 129 and use barrier methods of contraception.

It is also possible that if you overdo the progesterone cream, if you are using it when it is not appropriate to your needs, or if you are one of the small number of sensitive individuals who find that it does not agree with them, you may have side effects from using it. This is usually felt as tissue bloating, especially around the legs and ankles or breasts. If you experience this, or any other adverse symptoms, stop taking the natural progesterone, or experiment with a lower dose during your next cycle.

You can certainly overdose on natural progesterone, as you can on anything. However, it is a hormone which is made in the body in milligrams, which is a huge amount when compared to the nanograms of all other hormones, at least pre-menopausally.

WHAT IS NATURAL ABOUT TAKING PROGESTERONE?

In her book about natural HRT Marilyn Glenville poses the question 'What is so "natural" about the idea of women taking progesterone?' And she does have a point. After the menopause our bodies do not make progesterone in significant quantities, which does beg the question why we should be taking it at that time. It is all a matter of perspective and, as I describe in **Progesterone and the Menopause** on page 158, perhaps our current average lifespan is not in accord with our biological clock. There is no doubt in my mind that the most important factors to consider are diet and attention to vitamin and mineral levels, which in this day and age of reduced vitality of foods may mean taking supplements. Marilyn Glenville is right in making the point that the starting point for progesterone and oestrogen manufacture is cholesterol, which suggests that what is important is correcting dietary and lifestyle factors to encourage accurate levels of hormones from the building materials. But the reality is that many women are now affected by severe hormonal imbalance problems pre-menopausally, such as endometriosis and polycystic ovaries, which may need more than adjustments to diet to resolve them in the long run. And post-menopausally the information regarding natural progesterone and osteoporosis looks extremely positive. If a person is inclined to consider hormone replacement then the natural alternatives seem to beat the pharmaceutical preparations on many counts. It is really a personal call.

NATURAL OESTROGEN

To re-cap, there are three main types of oestrogen, E1, E2 and E3. The first two are 'strong' oestrogens which have been linked, in excess, to conditions such as endometriosis, breast and uterine cancers. The last one, E3, is considered benign and not involved in any detrimental health problems. Oestrogen supplementation is not needed as often as progesterone supplementation. Successful effects can be achieved by eating foods which are rich in phytoestrogens, or by using phytoestrogenic herbs, rather than supplementing oestrogens directly. This is why it is generally helpful to add soya and other phytoestrogen-rich foods into your diet on a regular basis. By eating these foods you can help to balance out your own oestrogen levels – dampen down excess if it exists, and supplement levels if they are declining.

There are some cases where it may be helpful to use oestrogen cream, which is in the form of the milder, benign, E3 oestriol. Your GP may advise you to use it if you have hot flushes which resist improvement through use of progesterone alone, or for vaginal dryness. In the case of vaginal dryness you can rub oestriol cream directly on to the area.

Using oestrogens is not advised if you have varicose veins, high blood pressure, diabetes, elevated blood fat levels, fibrocystic breasts, fibroids, are seriously overweight, have a family history of breast, endometrial or ovarian cancers, or have any clotting disorders.

FIND A FRIENDLY GP

All hormones are powerful chemicals and are not to be used lightly. Even natural ones, used to excess or at the wrong times, can have undesired effects. They must be used wisely and preferably under knowledgeable supervision. Natural hormones are available by prescription, but many GPs are not familiar with their use as they are trained in the use of synthetic hormones and not natural ones. You may even find that, as a result, your GP refuses to prescribe natural hormones. There are some GPs who are practised in their use and a list of them, with their addresses, is available – see the **Resources** section. These hormones can also be obtained by mail order for your own personal use, however it is best to find a GP who is familiar with them to advise and monitor their use. I would not advise self-prescribing any hormones. This is even more important if you have been diagnosed with any of the female hormone cancers.

TESTING HORMONE LEVELS

If you plan to use natural hormones, it may be wise to have an annual test of your hormone levels. You can have a blood test for progesterone levels carried out at your GP's surgery, though this may not be sensitive enough. The test can tell you if you are having anovulatory cycles (when you do not produce any progesterone in the latter half of the cycle), and also whether you are heading towards the menopause.

Of more use, in the context of using natural hormones, is the saliva test. This is available from doctors and nutritional therapists trained in its use. The saliva test is a more sensitive test for progesterone levels, but it can only be carried out privately (see **Resources**).

Unfortunately, there is no available test to tell you about exposure to xenoestrogens and the impact they may be having on your body. At best, you can only guess at the situation by working out if your exposure is high and if you have any symptoms.

Part Five

TARGETING

HEALTH

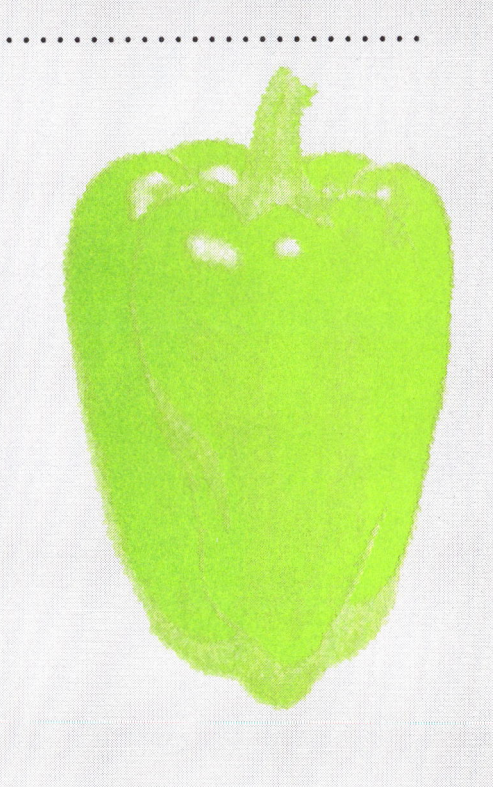

CHAPTER TWELVE

Introduction

Putting the 7-Point Plan into practice will go a long way towards resolving many hormone balance problems, especially when combined with avoiding xenoestrogens, and possibly experimenting with herbal remedies or natural hormones to see if they achieve the desired results. However, there may be specific problems which you would like to address, and in this chapter we will review the most common of the hormone-related ailments, with pointers about how to manage them.

CHAPTER THIRTEEN

Balancing Blood Sugar Levels

We have already reviewed blood sugar balance in relation to female hormone balance. Here we will investigate the most appropriate steps to take to restore even levels. Following the 7-Point Plan will take you the majority of the way, but some extra information may be useful.

As a general rule, carbohydrates which are whole and in their original form are less likely to be those which trigger blood sugar imbalance. For instance, a baked potato with the skin intact will give better blood sugar levels for sustained energy and hormone balance, whereas mashed potato or, even worse, packet mashed potato will send blood sugar levels soaring. It is usually the case that processed foods are high in refined carbohydrates and sugars which will have a detrimental effect on overall hormone balance. We take in 80 per cent of the 50kg of sugar we eat annually per person from packaged foods and not from the sugar bowl.

Foods are graded on a scale called the Glycaemic Index, which measures the speed with which foods are broken down to release sugars into the bloodstream. They are measured against glucose, which is given a score of 100, as it is the sugar found in blood. If we eat glucose, it passes into our blood immediately without being digested or metabolised. Foods which score 70–100 are best limited dramatically, while foods which score 50–70 are best eaten in moderation. Foods which score under 50 can be eaten freely by those with blood sugar problems.

In addition to this, it is helpful to eat little and often. This does not necessarily mean eating more in terms of quantity, but dividing up meals so that you manage a snack mid-morning and mid-afternoon, to keep blood sugar levels constant. The trick is to eat something before you get hungry, which is the time when you are most likely to reach for the sugary snacks. Ideal snacks include a piece of fruit, a plain yoghurt, a handful of fresh nuts or seeds (perhaps mixed in with a little dried fruit if you crave sweetness), a cup of vegetable soup, a wholegrain cracker with a little hummus or mackerel paté or an oatcake with a little cottage cheese. Most of these snacks also have the advantage of including some protein, which helps to regulate the impact that the carbohydrates have on blood sugar balance.

Eating a diet high in fibre is of prime importance in stabilising blood sugar levels and whole grains, pulses, vegetables and fruit are the best sources of dietary fibre. Supplemented fibre, in the form, for instance, of linseeds, psyllium husks, oat or rice bran can also contribute to blood sugar balance.

Once you have got into the habit of eating foods which help to stabilise blood sugar levels, you can then concentrate on reducing those which contribute to the problem, particularly sugar, alcohol and stimulants such as coffee and strong tea. You may also need to dilute fruit juices with at least 50 per cent water as they do not have any fibre to slow down the impact on blood sugar. Avoid eating handfuls of dried fruit, though it is fine to have a few dried fruits chopped up in yoghurts, with cereal or with nuts and seeds, but they can be too sugary on their own if you have blood sugar problems.

Exercise also helps to balance blood sugar levels, and has an effect on balancing all the other hormones needed for female hormone balance. Two to four hours a week is the recommended level.

Supplements which can help blood sugar control include:

- **Chromium** 200–500 mcg daily. The dose is weight dependent – in other words if you are heavy take a higher dose, and vice versa. Chromium is best taken alongside a B-complex, 50mg daily, as the B3 and B6 in the B-complex helps the chromium to work more effectively. (If you are an insulin-dependent diabetic, introduce chromium very slowly, while having your insulin intake monitored by your doctor, because chromium makes insulin work even more efficiently, meaning you may be able to reduce your insulin dose. This is best undertaken with the help of a qualified nutritionist.) Sources of chromium include wholegrains, brewer's yeast, shellfish, chicken, liver, eggs, mushrooms, milk, butter, bananas, carrots, cabbages, oranges, lettuce, apples, parsnips and potatoes.
- **Magnesium** is another important blood sugar balancing mineral and at levels of 200–300 mg per day can make a significant impact. Magnesium can be found in all green leafy vegetables, nuts, seeds, raisins, figs, garlic, onions, potatoes, chicken, yellow corn, aubergines and tomatoes.
- **Liquorice DGL** (deglycyrrhizinated). While liquorice is extremely useful for helping to balance blood sugar levels this supplement should not be taken if you have high blood pressure as it affects sodium/potassium balance.
- **Alpha-lipoic acid**, an antioxidant, has been shown to be very beneficial at stabilising blood sugar levels in diabetics at doses of 300–500 mg.

Glycaemic Index

G.I. Range: 15–50 ENJOY
Durum pasta, tortilla, wholewheat spaghetti, brown rice
Most fruits, dried apricots, dried apples
Fruit juices (best diluted 50/50 with water)
Beans, lentils, pulses, peas
High bran cereals, porridge
Most vegetables
Dairy foods
70 per cent cocoa solids dark chocolate (check labels as most are 30 per cent)
Fructose sugar, FOS sugar

G.I. Range: 50–70 LIMIT
Watermelon, bananas, potatoes with skin
Muesli, many plain biscuits
Rye crispbread, wholemeal bread, oatcakes
Most dried fruit, jam
Couscous

G.I. Range: 70–100 AVOID
Glucose, maltose, sugar, honey
White bread, white rice, rice cakes
Cornflakes, rice puffs
Cooked parsnips, carrots, beets
French fries, mashed potato
Water crackers
Colas and similar soft drinks
Milk chocolate, sweet biscuits
Alcohol

Closely linked to blood sugar balance is the question of adrenal health. The dietary suggestions for those who feel that they have been under chronic pressure, sufficient to impact upon their adrenal function, are very similar to those suggested for managing blood sugar levels. There are additional supplements, however, which can help adrenal function, and these include:

- **Vitamin C** is the ultimate stress nutrient and is used up in huge quantities when we are under any kind of stress, mental, physical, emotional or environmental. Animals manufacture it in abundance when they are under stress but we have lost that facility. Three grams a day has been shown to reduce the effects of adrenaline and can be highly supportive by protecting your body tissues against the ravages of stress.
- **The B-complex**, and in particular B5 and B6, are needed for the production of stress hormones. They are also involved in energy production in each and every cell. A 50-mg or 100-mg B-complex is an important supplement to protect against stress. You will probably find that your urine turns bright yellow as a result of the B2, but this is perfectly all right.
- **Zinc and magnesium**, which are the main stress minerals. Taking around 25 mg daily of zinc, and 300 mg daily of magnesium can be highly protective. Zinc is needed for all growth and repair jobs in the body, and can be depleted when people are under stress. This is one reason why skin, nails and hair show the effects of stress. Magnesium is essential for 300 processes in the body, and the stress process uses up large amounts.
- **Various herbs** are termed 'adaptogenic'. This means that they can help the body to adapt to stress. Different herbs

work in various ways either directly helping to stop active hormones from converting into inactive hormones or by influencing the feedback response of the hypothalamus. The ginsengs are all useful adaptogens. Korean ginseng is the most stimulating, Siberian ginseng slightly less so, while American ginseng is the most calming.

CHAPTER FOURTEEN

Boosting Your Thyroid

If you have been diagnosed with a low thyroid function by your doctor, the following can help to improve thyroid function. If you have not got sufficiently low thyroid function for it to show up on tests run by your doctor, it is still possible that you have a 'sub-clinically' under-performing thyroid. This is most evident when your body temperature is regularly on the low side, as described previously.

The most important measure is, once again, to reduce sugar levels, alcohol, caffeine and dependency on foods to which you may be sensitive, and certainly those to which you are addicted. Follow the advice in **Balancing Blood Sugar Levels** on page 104.

The most likely culprit, in terms of food sensitivities affecting the thyroid, is wheat. If you think that you may be sensitive to wheat, have a trial period without eating it to see if your health improves. Wheat can be particularly disruptive to the thyroid gland. Foods to avoid during a two-week phase include bread, pasta, pastry, biscuits, cake and any foods which list starch on the ingredients list. Instead use alternative grains and foods such as oatcakes, rye crackers, rice cakes, porridge, buckwheat noodles, corn, pasta, rice, quinoa and millet.

If you have very low thyroid function, then you may also want to limit the cruciferous family of vegetables to no more than three helpings a week. The cruciferous family include: broccoli, cauliflower, cabbage, Brussels sprouts and kale. However, these vegetables are excellent for overall health, so do not restrict them too much, and make sure that you get plenty of vegetables from other sources. Excessive soya may also inter-

fere with thyroid function, so you may want to limit it
times a week as well, and compensate by eating more

Seaweed is high in iodine and selenium, minerals needed for thyroid health, as well as being a rich source of calcium and potassium and many other trace minerals. You can buy seaweed in grinders to use like salt as a condiment, which adds a pleasant taste to savoury dishes, soups and salads. You could also supplement these minerals by taking a multi-mineral tablet daily, using kelp supplements or using a 'green-food' supplement with algae, spirulina, green wheat and other green foods. Important minerals for thyroid function are zinc and selenium, which help to turn the inactive hormone into the active form. Selenium-rich foods are Brazil nuts (two a day gives a therapeutic dose of selenium), seafood and fish, tomatoes, broccoli, rice, wholegrains and brewer's yeast. If you think you need a supplemental boost, you can take 25 mg daily of zinc and 200 mcg daily of selenium. Do not be tempted to take higher doses, especially of selenium, which can be toxic at high levels. Very rarely zinc makes people feel nauseous, in which case make sure you take the supplement with your food, and if this does not resolve the problem, try another brand, or stop using it altogether.

One of the classic signs of an underactive thyroid is bloating. Low thyroid hormone levels upset the balance of sodium and potassium, which leads to water retention. Eating lots of potassium-rich foods such as fruits and vegetables will help with this problem.

Remember that progesterone enhances thyroid hormone activity and if you are using it you may need to cut back on your thyroid medication (with your doctor's approval).

Again, overall health will always benefit from exercise – it significantly improves metabolism, and if you feel that you have a sluggish metabolism, then exercise should be a great boon.

CHAPTER FIFTEEN

Thrush and Cystitis

These two problems frequently plague women with hormone imbalance, or those who have been using the contraceptive pill for a while. They can be persistent and very uncomfortable. Frequently they are triggered by taking courses of antibiotics and steroid medication, as well as the Pill.

Thrush, or candida, is an infection of the vagina and surrounding area and the main symptoms are a thick white discharge and itchiness. It is usually caused by the yeast *candida albicans*, and quite often recurs until it is properly brought under control. The most common medication is an anti-thrush medication such as Canesten, but this usually only gets rid of the problem for a short while. It frequently takes a combination of diet and anti-thrush medication or supplements to really make sure that the infection does not recur. Thrush is frequently brought on by pregnancy, and many women will fail to tell the pharmacist that they are pregnant. Anti-thrush medication is not advised while pregnant.

Candida responds well to dietary changes, but if it is difficult to shift, it may turn out to be trichomoniasis – a protozoa parasite infection, in which case your doctor may recommend a drug such as Flagyl.

Cystitis is an inflammation of the bladder and the urethra, which is the tube leading out of the bladder through which urine passes. It is usually caused by infection with bacteria, often E.coli. It can also develop as an allergic reaction to scented bath products, and can be exacerbated by sexual activity, stress and food sensitivities. The main symptom is a stinging sensation when needing to urinate. The usual treatment is with antibiotics, if it is bacteria related, but this often means that the problem recurs as the bacteria become resistant to later courses of antibiotics. Antibiotics are also quite likely to act as a trigger for thrush.

Dietary treatment for both conditions centres on eliminating all refined carbohydrates, particularly sugar, alcohol and white flour products. Other sugary foods such as undiluted fruit juices and dried fruit also need to be limited drastically for a while. It may also be necessary to avoid foods which are sources of yeast, instead use unleavened breads such as soda bread, scones, oatcakes, pitta breads and rye crackers (though check the ingredients lists on the packages first). Beware of yeast in blue, hard and soft cheeses (but not curds such as cottage cheese), alcohol, vinegars and mushrooms (including Quorn). Severe cases may need to follow a proper anti-candida diet such as the one described in *Banish Bloating* in this series of books. The other major dietary step is to avoid foods to which you think you may be sensitive. Highest on the likely hit-list are wheat and dairy produce.

Eat a wholefood diet with plenty of vegetables, wholegrains, soya, pulses, lean meats and fresh fruit. Also make sure that you drink lots of water – two litres daily. Supporting your immune system is vital to help it to fight infections. Avoid coffee and strong tea, and other stimulants which have the effect of suppressing the immune system. Fruits and vegetables contain the vital antioxidants which support immune function and help to keep yeast infections and cystitis at bay. The most important fruits are the berries such as blackberries, strawberries, blueberries and raspberries, as they are rich in antioxidants called proanthocyanidins which are potent immune supporters. Eating garlic, olive oil and live yoghurt are delicious ways to enhance immune health and to control yeast infections.

Supplements can help as well, and taking an antioxidant supplement daily can help to support your immune system. Selenium is essential for the immune system, as are the antioxidant vitamins A, C and E. Taking a daily supplement which gives 200 mcg of selenium, at least 100 ius of vitamin E and 7,500 ius of vitamin A can be a great help. Vitamin A is also necessary for the health of the urinary tract and vaginal mucus membranes. Acidophilus, which is a beneficial bacteria, helps to control both thrush and cystitis infections and if you do not eat live yoghurt daily, supplement with some beneficial bacteria capsules. You can also supplement garlic – if you are unable to eat one clove a day, take supplements to give 10 mg of allium daily.

Tips to help deal with a cystitis crisis:

- For an acute cystitis infection, drink two litres of unsweetened cranberry juice a day until the cystitis goes, or take cranberry supplements. Cranberries reduce the adherence of bacteria to the walls of the urethra and bladder. Juniper berries also have a similar action, as do blueberries.
- Drink a half a litre of water when an attack of cystitis starts and carry on drinking the same amount every 20 minutes afterwards. Every hour stir a teaspoon of bicarbonate of soda into the water. Keep up this regime for three hours.
- Alternatively, combine two teaspoons of apple cider vinegar with one cup of water, and sweeten with honey. Drink one cup three times daily.
- If you have cystitis also take a gram of vitamin C, with bioflavanoids, every couple of hours until the infection subsides. The vitamin C is excreted in the urine, which means that it gets to the 'parts that really need it'.

- 200 mg of magnesium citrate makes the urine more alkaline, which reduces problems with cystitis.
- Uva ursi, also known as bearberry, is a herb which is very useful for dealing with a cystitis crisis. It takes longer than antibiotics to work, but it is effective and does not have the drawback that antibiotics can have of creating resistance. Uva ursi is also useful for E.coli infections. Take 1–4 grams of dried leaf equivalent three times daily for seven days. Do not overuse as it can cause nausea in high amounts (also do not take if pregnant or breastfeeding). If cystitis persists, however, it is important to have your doctor check it, as the infection can travel up towards the kidneys and turn into a more serious infection.

Tips to help deal with a thrush crisis:

- A pessary of a peeled garlic clove inserted in the vagina can help to get rid of a yeast infection. Whatever you do, make sure that the garlic clove is not cut in any way or you will find the burning sensation very uncomfortable.
- A douche of the vaginal area twice daily with warm water into which a few drops of tea-tree oil has been added. Alternatively, a douche of 2 tbsp of apple cider vinegar to a litre of warm water used twice daily is helpful. You can also add three or four drops of grapefruit seed extract to this douche.
- Another, more messy, but very effective douche is made with 25 grams of plain, live yoghurt, 1 tsp of raw (not pasteurised) honey and 1 tbsp of aloe vera gel or juice.
- Taking oregano oil supplements is highly effective against yeast, and is thought to be many times more effective than the more frequently used supplement caprylic acid. Take

0.6 mg in two or three divided doses daily (but not if pregnant or breastfeeding).
- Goldenseal, the active component of which is berberine, is a highly effective anti-microbial. It is useful against both yeast and cystitis infections. Take 1–2 grams dried root/rhizome equivalent three times daily (but not if pregnant or breastfeeding).

CHAPTER SIXTEEN

Moontime Madness

> The monthly activity of the ovaries . . . may become
> an important cause of mental and physical derangement.
> *Henry Maudsley*, psychiatrist, 1873

It has been suggested that as many as 80 per cent of women of childbearing age experience PMS. PMS is defined as persistent symptoms which recur prior to menstruation and last anything from one day to two weeks. These symptoms can include: bloating and weight gain, mood swings, irregular cycles, tension, headaches, anxiety, irritability, sugar cravings, aggression, depression, weepiness, a lack of self-esteem, feelings of helplessness, insomnia, change in sex drive, skin eruptions, water retention, palpitations, back pain, cold symptoms. No wonder women might have been convinced in earlier times that they were indeed going mad!

Severe PMS is called Premenstrual Dysphoric Disorder (PMDD). It is to be applauded that the medical profession now recognises that such a phenomenon exists, as previously it was suggested that such problems were often all in the woman's mind. However, it is a little sad that there is still such a strong emphasis on medicating it – the antidepressant Prozac is now licensed for use for severe PMDD and no doubt other similar medications will follow – rather than looking at ways of preventing the problem.

Four types of PMS have been identified by Maryon Stewart of The Women's Nutritional Advisory Service – the ABCD of premenstrual problems:

A – ANXIETY: Symptoms include nervous tension, irritability, mood swings and anxiety. These symptoms can become progressively worse as the period nears. It is believed that rising oestrogen levels predispose some women to this. If the liver is not processing oestrogens properly and re-circulating them back into the blood, levels of oestrogen can be abnormally high. Factors which influence this include a lack of B-vitamins, which are involved in the liver's handling of oestrogens, and a low fibre-high fat diet. B-vitamins, along with magnesium, are needed for normal production of the brain chemical dopamine. A disturbed balance of dopamine can lead to anxiety. Caffeine has also been implicated, as side effects include anxiety, irritability, depression, headaches and dehydration.

B – BLOATING: Water retention can affect all parts of the body premenstrually, but particularly the breasts, the hands, the feet, the ankles, the abdomen and waistline. While they may feel very bloated, usually only 1–2 kg is gained in actual weight. Occasionally it is more than this and can be as much as 2.5–5kg. Generally the factors associated with this kind of premenstrual strife are the same as for the 'anxiety' type, with high oestrogen levels being the main factor. Salt is another factor in water retention and cutting back on salty and packaged foods, as well as the salt cellar, can help.

C – CRAVINGS: Cravings for particular foods, especially carbohydrates, sugars and stimulants can take on overwhelming proportions in the days or two weeks before a period. This situation is described in full in the chapter **Balancing Blood Sugar Levels**, page 104, and relates to the interaction between female hormones, blood sugar hormones and adrenaline. This is a vicious cycle as the foods which are craved often lead to a variety of other symptoms, including all of the other three types of PMS – bloating, anxiety and depression. It is also possible that women crave more carbohydrates, or other foods, at this time, and any borderline food sensitivities can develop into more serious symptoms premenstrually. This is particularly the case with sugar, dairy products, wheat, alcohol, coffee and chocolate, and these can lead to more bloating symptoms.

D – DEPRESSION: This usually occurs alongside other types of premenstrual problems, especially the Anxiety type. The contributing factors are not fully known, but diet does improve a number of cases where clinical depression does not exist. B-vitamins can certainly help, as can reducing dependency on stimulants. Levels of a brain chemical, serotonin, are affected by oestrogen levels and this would explain why the antidepressant drug Prozac is now being used successfully in some cases.

HIGH PROGESTERONE PMS

While around 70 per cent of women who suffer PMS have too much oestrogen premenstrually, about 30 per cent of women have the reverse – too much progesterone, and too little natural oestrogen. It is also possible to have both high oestrogen and high progesterone at the same time. No solid research is available about the specific impact of xenoestrogens on these groups, but they are suspected of contributing to the problem as they seem to with most other hormone driven symptoms.

These different types of premenstrual hormone imbalance explain why natural progesterone can help so many women premenstrually (those with high oestrogen), but also why others (those with high progesterone) find their symptoms exacerbated by natural progesterone, in which case stop using it immediately. It is possible to have your hormone levels checked (see **Natural Hormones** page 98).

HEAVY PERIODS

We all have a different experience with quantity of flow, but for some women the scale of bleeding each month can be a cause for alarm. This is especially the case if there is a significant change in the amount of flow from what you would consider normal. An increase in flow can signal fibroids in the womb or endometriosis so, if you are concerned, it is wise to have a check-up. See the sections on **Fibroids** and **Endometriosis** on pages 139 and 140.

There is a possible link between low vitamin A levels and heavy blood loss. Vitamin A is stored in the liver, and blood levels, which are released from the liver, fluctuate throughout the cycle, probably correlating to hormone levels. Studies have shown that women with heavy periods have lower blood levels of vitamin A, and that treatment with a vitamin A supplement can improve the symptoms significantly or even provide complete relief. The contraceptive pill can create a high level of vitamin A in the blood by moving it out of storage in the liver, and thus women on the Pill tend to have an easy time with blood flow. Just after stopping the Pill it is common for women to experience a heavy flow. This may be linked to blood levels of vitamin A plummeting. Vitamin A works alongside vitamin E and zinc, and a lack of these nutrients can also masquerade as vitamin A deficiency so, when taking vitamin A, it is best to take the nutrients which work synergistically alongside it. Daily doses of 7,500–15,000 ius of vitamin A can help to replenish levels, but do not take vitamin A if you are planning a pregnancy or are pregnant. In this instance take an equivalent amount of beta-carotene, the water soluble pre-vitamin A.

Iron levels are often low as a result of heavy blood flow and if you are feeling tired and have pale skin, then it is wise to have your blood iron levels checked by your doctor. If you need to take an iron supplement, you may find that the type offered by your doctor, ferrous sulphate, has a constipating effect. If this happens you can use different, less-constipating, types of iron supplements such as ferrous gluconate, 10–20 mg daily (only take more than this if advised to by your doctor). Alternatively, you can take beetroot extract supplements which increase blood levels of iron more gently. You can also eat beetroot daily, in which case eat it raw. Raw beetroot is delicious, just wash it, peel it if you wish, grate or slice it and sprinkle with lemon juice. The best source of iron, if you are not a vegetarian, is red meat which provides highly absorbable haem iron. Also avoid using wheat bran, or bran-based cereals as the phytates they contain can impair iron absorption. Supplementing green foods such as spirulina and chlorella can also improve iron intake (see **Resources**).

Vitamin C, together with bioflavanoids, can help to control heavy periods. The bioflavanoids are the synergistic compounds found just below the skin of fruits and vegetables. Vitamin C is much more effective with these compounds. Eat a wide variety of fruit and vegetables, at least five portions daily, and take vitamin C supplements – 1 gram three times daily. Vitamin C also increases the absorption of iron from foods, so a small glass of orange juice with a meal can significantly help iron uptake as well as give you an extra quota of vitamin C, and this is very helpful for vegetarians who do not eat red meat.

The polyunsaturated fats found in evening primrose oil, starflower oil and borage oil can be particularly helpful if you have heavy periods with a tendency to clot. Read the package and take sufficient to give you 100–200 mg of the active compound GLA daily.

PERIOD CRAMPS

Any muscle can be susceptible to cramps, which indicate that they have trouble contracting and relaxing. The muscles of the womb are no different. During a period the muscles of the womb have to work hard to shed its inner lining, which we experience as blood loss, and this can be very uncomfortable for some women. Women who have not yet had a baby are more susceptible to painful periods.

The main foods which can adversely affect period cramps are red meat and dairy produce. They contain the type of fats which interfere with short-term hormones called prostaglandins, and this can encourage inflammation. On the other hand, the healthy fats from sources such as fish oils and polyunsaturated fats can improve the performance of anti-inflammatory prostaglandins. Caffeinated drinks and alcohol can also impact on muscle cramping by interfering with mineral absorption from the diet, exerting a diuretic effect and interfering with the conversion of the healthy fats we have just been discussing into anti-inflammatory prostaglandins.

The key nutrient which can help to reduce period cramps is magnesium. The minerals calcium and magnesium govern the working of nerves which regulate muscle contractions. Magnesium, which, according to Government figures, is deficient in the diet of 72 per cent of women, is not only directly responsible for a part of this process, but also helps the body to use calcium more effectively. Sources of calcium and magnesium include: dark green leafy vegetables, nuts, seeds, wholegrains, soya beans, legumes, dried fruit, sardines, salmon. Dairy products are a rich source of calcium but have very little magnesium which can serve to upset mineral balance.

All cramps, including leg cramps and 'fluttering' eyelids, can benefit from a diet high in magnesium and calcium, and the use of supplements if necessary. Start off with supplementing a ratio of 2 to 1 – for instance, 600 mg magnesium to 300 mg calcium daily. As your symptoms improve you can shift to a ratio of 1 to 1 – 600 mg magnesium to 600 mg calcium daily. Eventually you should be able to lower your dose or, if you wish, wean yourself off the supplements altogether.

Other supplements which can help period cramps are vitamin E (400–800 ius), zinc (25 mg) and evening primrose oil (100–200 mg GLA).

IRREGULAR PERIODS

It is necessary to define what an irregular period is. As we have already discussed, a normal cycle can be anything between 20 days and 40 days between periods. Periods can be skipped for no particular reason and, while you may want to check this with your doctor, it is not normally anything to worry about. You may, of course, also want to run a pregnancy test!

If the frequency of your periods starts to alter significantly, you may be moving towards the menopause. The menopause phase normally begins any time from the age of around 40 to 55. One in a hundred women have a very early menopause and this can occur as young as the age of 16, only two to four years after the onset of periods. For these young women this can be a confusing and upsetting time, and this is where hormonal treatment, in-vitro fertility treatment with egg donation, and wise counselling, can really come into their own.

Absent or irregular periods can also be associated with a number of other factors, including low body weight, anorexia nervosa, overtraining for sport, the contraceptive pill and extreme stress. Parents of daughters who stop menstruating and who have a very low body weight need to be alert to the possibility of anorexia. High stress levels can lead to both missed periods and to more frequent periods. If you are experiencing irregular periods it is even more important to follow the **7-Point Plan** and, if necessary, have your hormone levels checked by your doctor.

BLOATING

When there is an excess of oestrogen just prior to a period, or a deficiency of progesterone, the balance in favour of oestrogen encourages more water retention. These two factors can play havoc with bloating in the two days, or even two weeks, before the onset of a period.

Most women will be familiar with blood sugar irregularities premenstrually, suggesting that insulin control has gone out of the window having been triggered by oestrogen and progesterone imbalance. This is when your normal iron-will falls apart and you hoover up anything and everything sugary or starchy. Many women need more energy 'props' just before their period is due. Therefore, not only are the effects of excess oestrogen being felt, but the knock-on effect on blood sugar balance means that the bacteria in the bowels are feeding on all the sugary and starchy foods which are most likely to be implicated in water retention and digestive bloating. Foods to which you are addicted become irresistible and contribute to the bloating you are already experiencing.

If you are taking the contraceptive pill, and you find that you are experiencing bloating, this probably indicates that the oestrogen levels in the pill are too high for you. It is best to talk to your doctor about taking a lower-dose oestrogen pill or, even better, to stop taking the pill and find a natural alternative. This latter course of action will also mean that you will be more in tune with your body and able to monitor your hormone balance according to your symptoms. Dietary adjustments, such as those below, can make all the difference with balancing hormones.

DIET TO BANISH PMS

The measures described in the **7-Point Plan** will help to balance out hormone levels. The most important factors are cutting out sugar, caffeine and alcohol, increasing fibre levels, and reducing animal sources of fats and overall fat levels. Alongside this, pay attention to stress levels, and to thyroid health. It is helpful to eat organic food wherever possible to reduce exposure to environmental oestrogens.

Addressing any food allergies or sensitivities can have a profound effect on PMS, though this may be hard to distinguish from the daily symptoms experienced as a result of food-related problems. The most common are wheat and dairy sensitivities, but any foods can be implicated. Alternatives to wheat are given in Point 6 of the 7-Point Plan, but if you are avoiding dairy products you may want to experiment with some of the following: soya milk, soya yoghurt, rice milk, oat milk or coconut milk (diluted).

If you do not have an allergy problem with soya, eating it on a regular basis can have a balancing effect on oestrogens – 50–100 grams of tofu daily, or 1 1/2 (1/2 litre) glasses of soya milk daily can make a difference. You can also buy soya flour and soya flakes to add to baked products or to stews, salads, soups and casseroles. Breads are now being marketed called 'ladies' bread'. These are good sources of soya and linseeds which have a hormone balancing effect. Beans, which are good sources of fibre, are also fairly high in similar compounds to those contained in soya called phytoestrogens. These help to block body oestrogens from their bloating effects.

Foods rich in potassium can help to alleviate PMS and, in particular, the water retention associated with it. Bananas, tomatoes, watermelon (including the seeds) and potatoes are potassium rich, though all fruit and vegetables offer good amounts. Other potassium-rich foods include nuts and fish.

Some foods have a diuretic action and can be helpful if you experience water retention. Increase your intake of artichokes, asparagus, parsley, watercress and chamomile tea. Avoid salt as it encourages water retention. Drink two litres of water daily to keep your system hydrated and cleansed.

Supplemented nutrients can also help. Vitamin B6 encourages the correct processing of oestrogen through the liver, while the B-vitamins as a complex, and choline, which is found in lecithin, help to deactivate oestrogens in the liver. Apart from the B-vitamins, the most important nutrients to supplement are magnesium, vitamin E and GLA, in the form of evening primrose oil, starflower oil or borage oil. The order in which to tackle the problem is to address diet and exercise first, then add in supplements when you know what residual problems are left. If all else fails, you probably need to investigate whether a low-dose of thyroid hormone, or natural progesterone can help. Supplementing histadine – an amino acid – should be avoided as it can worsen the symptoms of PMS, probably because it is involved in histamine production which can increase inflammation.

Don't forget about exercise. Exercise has been proven to lower excess oestrogen levels in the body significantly, and can help to regulate overall hormone levels. The minimum amount which has a meaningful impact seems to be around an hour of exercise, four times a week, sufficient to get your heart rate up a bit, but not so much that you are out of breath and cannot hold a conversation. Build up slowly to this level if you are unused to exercise, and check with your doctor before embarking on a programme if you have cardiovascular problems.

MOOD SWINGS

The majority of mood swings can be resolved with blood sugar regulation (see **Balancing Blood Sugar Levels**, page 104). In really severe cases, however, it may need more attention to detail, and I have found it common for women to need a small snack every 1 1/2–2 hours to keep their blood sugar levels topped up. Appropriate snacks are low sugar, high complex carbohydrates and moderate proteins, as described in the section on blood sugar balance, page 107. Stimulants prompt sugar cravings and caffeine can encourage depression. Sugar, caffeine and alcohol also use up B-vitamins and decrease potassium, zinc and magnesium levels. Give coffee, strong tea and alcohol a miss for a while. Magnesium helps to maintain normal brain chemical metabolism and hormone balance, and yet it is deficient in around 50 per cent of women with PMS. Vitamin B6 can help premenstrually and 50–100 mg B-complex can go a long way in alleviating premenstrual problems, though it may be necessary to increase the dose to 200 mg premenstrually. B6 is needed to stimulate the manufacture of the amino acid tryptophan, which affects B3 production. B3 is needed to regulate blood sugar levels and is involved in the 'mood brain chemical' serotonin. This is why B6 and B3 can often help alleviate depression, sleep disturbances and headaches, all of which can be worse premenstrually.

High oestrogen to progesterone levels can result in low levels of the brain chemical serotonin, and also lowered endorphins in the brain. These lower levels can lead to a variety of symptoms, including the need to binge. They can affect moods, too. Endorphins can be raised with exercise, and acupuncture may also be very effective. Stress often lowers endorphin levels. Low oestrogen levels can induce low dopamine levels, another brain chemical. This can lead to symptoms of depression or confusion, particularly in the second half of the cycle or pre-menopausally.

The mineral magnesium is needed for dopamine to be effective, and supplementing it can help a wide range of mental symptoms. The herbal antidepressant St John's wort has also been shown to be effective in mild to moderate depression.

It is also not uncommon for women who find that diet does not fully address the problem of their altered moods to discover that they have an imbalance of metals, particularly an excess of the heavy metals lead and cadmium and an excess of copper. If your moods do not resolve themselves despite following the **7-Point Plan** it may be wise to consult a nutritional therapist who can run tests to see if you have an excess of heavy metals. See the **Resources** section page 178.

CHAPTER SEVENTEEN

Fertility

During their fertile years women have the remarkable possibility of creating a new life 13 times each year. The health of the egg (ovum) and the sperm are paramount to the health of a newly created foetus, and for it to develop into a healthy, bonny baby.

NATURAL FAMILY PLANNING

Natural family planning methods can be used for both planning a pregnancy and for avoiding pregnancy. Finding that window of opportunity to conceive when a healthy sperm, which lives for only three or four days, can meet a healthy egg, which will live for an even shorter 24 hours can be a bit of a hit-and-miss affair. The merit of natural family planning is that the foetus can start its life in an environment which is unencumbered by recent exposure to synthetic sources of hormones. If you have the opposite scenario in mind, and are aiming to avoid a pregnancy, natural family planning will allow you to remain free of synthetic sources of hormones for your own health.

If your cycle does not fit into the 28-day 'mould' then it can be difficult knowing exactly when an egg has been released. There are three methods of checking when you are ovulating:

- Checking your temperature: Just after ovulation a woman's body temperature rises by a minimum of 0.2 degrees centigrade because of the influence of the hormone progesterone. If your temperature does not rise at all, it is possible that you are experiencing an anovulatory cycle, when an egg is not matured and released, and therefore progesterone is not being made. For about two or three cycles you need to take your temperature daily to establish when it is that you ovulate. Once you know this you can restrict taking your temperature to the five days before your anticipated ovulation and the couple of days after.

- Checking your cervical mucus: As levels of oestrogen rise towards the time of ovulation, cervical mucus changes from being cloudy and sticky to being clear, watery and slippery. You can find information about organisations which teach this method in the **Resources** section. The pH of the mucus also becomes more alkaline, which is helpful to sperm.
- You can buy ovulation predictor kits from most pharmacies, which test for hCG hormone levels in your urine. This is probably the most convenient method, but it is subject to false readings and is best conducted alongside one of the other two methods above.

If you do not want to become pregnant, it is best not to rely on these methods 100 per cent. To be more safe, use a barrier method of contraception alongside your chosen method of ovulation prediction. If you are stopping contraception because you believe that you have gone through the menopause it is generally advised that you allow two clear years without a period if you are under the age of 50, and one clear year without a period if you are over the age of 50.

PREPARING FOR A HEALTHY PREGNANCY

There are several steps to take to give your baby the best possible chance of being conceived and of establishing him or her in a healthy environment. Most women start to think about their pregnancy when they have a positive test. Ideally, the time to start thinking about it is at least three months, and preferably six months, before you hope to conceive. As I have already mentioned, all the eggs a woman needs for her reproductive life are in place while she is a foetus. Several million eggs are created and lie dormant. But not all of these eggs survive, and by the time a young woman starts to menstruate only around 300,000 of these eggs remain. It makes sense to ensure that these eggs are as healthy as possible so they can result in a successful pregnancy and, the ultimate aim, a healthy baby.

Here is a checklist of steps to take:

Six months to conception

- Stop taking the contraceptive pill if you are using it, and start using natural family planning methods.
- Have yourself, and your partner, tested and, if necessary, treated for chlamydia and other sexually transmitted diseases (STDs). For this you will need to visit your doctor or genito-urinary clinic. Infections can fundamentally affect the foetus and be responsible for early miscarriages and congenital defects. Chlamydia is the most common STD. It is frequently dormant and symptom free, but probably affects one in 14 sexually active people. If you have fertility problems it is one of the first things which should be checked for.
- Both you and your partner need to stop smoking.
- Start following a wholefood diet as outlined in the 7-Point Plan, and eat organic food if possible.

Three months to conception

- Start taking a pre-conceptual vitamin and mineral supplement which includes 400 mcg of folic acid, and which

sources its vitamin A from beta-carotene (stop taking any preparations with vitamin A in them). Avoid taking any herbal preparations unless you consult a qualified herbalist.
- Reduce your alcohol intake to the bare minimum, but certainly no more than four measures per week.

One month to conception
- Avoid all alcohol.
- Avoid all over-the-counter drugs. Speak to your doctor about stopping or reducing any prescribed medication (do not stop any prescribed medication without your doctor's consent).
- Continue to take your pre-conceptual vitamins and minerals up to and throughout the pregnancy.

INFERTILITY

It is quite common for a successful fertilisation to take from six to 18 months from the point that you start 'trying' for a family. If it takes longer than this then your doctor will be willing to do some tests to discover the possible reasons why you might not be conceiving. Sixty per cent of infertility cases can be traced back to the woman, 40 per cent to the man. There are a number of reasons why a woman may be experiencing problems conceiving and one important factor to rule out is a structural fault such as blocked fallopian tubes. Conditions such as endometriosis, infections and pelvic inflammatory disease can all contribute to infertility. Weight of the mother-to-be can also have a bearing on her likelihood of conceiving, with seriously underweight women having a greater risk of problems.

Nutrition can play a major part in resolving difficulties with conception by readying the woman's body, helping to change the acidity of the vaginal mucus to make it more receptive to sperm, reducing the impact of any environmental chemicals or heavy metals, and eliminating inflammatory diseases.

Certain nutrients are needed in abundance for a healthy pregnancy to be initiated and these include zinc, magnesium and essential fats. For more information about nutrition during pregnancy, read *Perfect Pregnancy* in this series of books.

HEALTHY SPERM

In the last 50 years, male sperm count has dropped from an average of 113 million per ml to an average of 66 million per ml. A sperm count of 20 million per ml is associated with infertility.

If planning a pregnancy, or if infertility is suspected, it is just as important to examine the man's role in what is going on. Sperm is created in the testes about three months before it is ejaculated, and to ensure the healthiest possible sperm it is best for men to do some pre-conceptual planning for four to six months before anticipated conception. Factors which affect the quality, quantity and motility of sperm include:

- Alcohol and smoking, both of which have an adverse effect on sperm production.
- Drugs – recreational and over-the-counter. You should check with your doctor about reducing or stopping any prescribed medication.
- Eating a healthy diet along the lines of the **7-Point Plan** on page 35.
- Avoiding sources of xenoestrogens for men is just as important as it is for women. Xenoestrogens have been implicated in lowered sperm production and various reproductive organ abnormalities in male babies. Particularly at risk are men who work in agriculture, as

livestock or dairy farmers, or fruit and flower growers, because of their high exposure to these chemicals.
- Particular nutrients are important for healthy sperm production and they include the minerals zinc and magnesium and the essential fats.
- For four to six months the man can greatly benefit if he takes a general multi-vitamin and mineral supplement, making sure that he gets 25mg of zinc, and 300 mg of magnesium. Eating foods rich in essential fats, including oily fish, fresh nuts and seeds, and dressing salads with cold-pressed walnut or flax oil is also beneficial.

CHAPTER EIGHTEEN

Bosom Buddies

Breast tissue is particularly responsive to the monthly swings of female hormones, and most women are acutely aware of this fact in the few days, or even the two weeks, before their period. The cells which make up the breasts have receptor sites for both oestrogen and progesterone. Just before a period many women have high enough levels of oestrogen to cause tissue swelling and discomfort.

If this were all there was to it, it might be acceptable to just 'put up and shut up'. But there is more involved here, with potentially worrying consequences. Oestrogens encourage sensitive cells to multiply more speedily, and this means that women can also be susceptible to lumps and bumps of different types. This, in itself, is still not hugely worrying, though it can cause a lot of distress as women may wonder if it is something more serious.

It is important to check breasts each month for any lumps or other irregularities which may be a sign of trouble. If you are pre-menopausal it is best to check your breasts a few days after your period, once your breasts have settled down. If you are post-menopausal, pick a convenient day each month when you can remember to do a check – say the first of the month. If you have had a hysterectomy which has left your ovaries intact, you may still be subject to hormonal swings and you will have to gauge a day, on a monthly basis, when your breasts are quiescent.

Eighty per cent of all lumps are found not to be cancerous and, generally speaking, if you are pre-menopausal the chances are much slimmer that any lump you find is cancerous.

However, it is important not to be complacent, as any suspicious change to the breast tissue and area surrounding it should be investigated by your doctor as soon as possible.

It is not always a lump you are looking for, but a change which is significantly different for you. Check under your armpits and over your collar-bone as well. Signs of breast cancer can include lumps, puckering skin, newly inverted nipples, discharge from the nipples (especially if one sided), eczema on the breast tissue, inflammation, bruising, or other changes.

Lumps and bumps can have a number of causes. Fibrocystic breast disease – general lumpiness – is so common these days that some physicians believe that it should not be identified as a disease. While the disease does not seem to increase the risk of breast cancer, it shares some of the same probable causes. Fibrocystic breast disease is thought to be due to high oestrogen levels and increased levels of prolactin (the breast milk hormone). It is also thought that in many women this can be the result of low thyroid hormone levels leading to high oestrogen, and then in turn to high prolactin. Sometimes lumps can be painful, sometimes not. Lumps can also be benign fibroadenomas, fat necrosis (lumps of dead fat tissue), or fluid-filled cysts.

Breast tenderness can be affected by the oestrogens in the contraceptive pill or HRT, and if you are on these preparations and believe that they are contributing to breast swelling and tenderness, or lumps, it is probably wise to stop taking them as it means that your breast tissue is overly sensitive to the oestrogens.

As I have mentioned, in 20 per cent of cases lumps do turn out to be cancerous, which is where the problem of excess oestrogens takes a very serious turn. The problem with cells dividing quickly is that a proportion of them will not have enough time to divide accurately, and this can lead to incorrectly 'programmed' cells. These rogue cells are, in the normal course of events, seen as interlopers and are cleaned up by the body's housekeeping mechanisms. But once in a while a badly programmed cell gets through the net and begins to divide out of control under the influence of oestrogens, and this can be the beginning of breast cancer.

As we have seen an increase of breast cancer incidence of 40 per cent in the last 30 years, it is important to address issues of oestrogen overload at an earlier, rather than a later, stage of a woman's life. Uncomfortably swollen breasts premenstrually are a sign that excessive oestrogens, or unopposed oestrogens, could well be a problem.

HEALTHY BREASTS

The management of breast swelling, discomfort and non-malignant lumps involves balancing hormones and this is covered in the 7-Point Plan for Hormone Health on page 35. In addition to the Plan, there are several other factors which can help to dramatically improve premenstrual breast discomfort.

Addressing food allergies is a step which reaps significant rewards for many women. The worst offenders are wheat, dairy products, other gluten grains such as rye, oats and barley, and, in some cases, soya products (even though soya helps by far the majority of women). These foods may be contributing to the problem because of impaired digestion leading to a build-up of fluids and fluid retention, which can be particularly painful in the breasts.

Caffeine can make fibrocystic breast disease worse for a number of women. Cutting out all sources of caffeine for three months is a worthwhile experiment. Sources include coffee, tea, colas, chocolate, guarana, headache medications and cold remedies. It is necessary to be rigorous about avoiding caffeine, as cutting back is not usually effective. You may also find that decaffeinated coffee is not useful as it also contains other compounds.

Caffeine, theobromine and theophylline together make up the methylxanthenes and the last two are even found in decaffeinated coffee, and all of these can be a problem. There are many coffee alternatives made from barley, dandelion or chicory, and a wide selection of refreshing herbal teas.

Women who exercise report considerably fewer problems with breast tenderness premenstrually, probably because of the effect of exercise in helping to eliminate oestrogens.

Certain nutrients are known to be effective at reducing the impact of premenstrual breast problems. Evening primrose oil, starflower oil or borage oil supplements which give 100–200 mg of the active compound GLA daily can help a number of women (very rarely GLA makes the swelling worse, which suggests that too much of this 'family' of fats is being consumed, and that more fish oil/flax oil fats are needed – see Point 1 in the 7-Point Plan). After this helpful oil, the next most likely nutrients are magnesium (300–400 mg daily) and vitamin B6 (100–200 mg daily). Vitamin E at levels of 800 ius can make a difference to some women, though it is important to persevere for at least three cycles to see if it has any impact. Do not take vitamin E without professional advice if you are taking blood-thinning medication such as Warfarin. Vitamin B1 (100 mg) can also help some women. Some phytoestrogenic herbal preparations can be helpful, refer to **Herbs For Harmony** on page 85, as can ginkgo biloba since it improves circulation and helps to keep breast tissue cleansed.

If you find that following the 7-Point Plan for at least three cycles does not resolve the problems you are experiencing, you may want to investigate your thyroid function. This can greatly help to impact on breast swelling and discomfort and low-dose thyroxine can benefit those who have low thyroid problems accompanied by breast symptoms. You may also want to experiment with natural progesterone. This option is covered in **Natural Hormones** on page 91.

CHAPTER NINETEEN

What's Up Down Under

The female reproductive tract can be afflicted with a number of disorders, all of which suggest hormonal or nutritional imbalances. In this chapter we will look at the most common problems.

Many of these diseases have, in the last few decades, shown a steady increase in incidence in developed countries. Painful heavy periods, endometriosis, pelvic inflammatory disease, fibroids – all of these are on the increase. Cancers of the cervix, ovaries and endometrium (uterine lining) are all rising, with these three cancers representing eight per cent of all diagnosed cancers annually.

FIBROIDS

Fibroids are benign lumps that grow attached to the muscular wall of the womb. They are firm and round and can vary from the size of a pea to that of a grapefruit, though it is when they reach the size of an apple that they seem to cause sufficient disruption to be investigated. They are strictly a hormonal problem, which is evident as they disappear after the menopause when oestrogen levels drop. In the meantime they can cause problems with excessive bleeding, due to the increased surface area of the womb lining, and the weight of them can be sufficient to weaken pelvic floor muscles leading to prolapses and stress incontinence (an involuntary loss of urine due to weakness of the relevant muscles). Surgery is often performed, either to remove the fibroids or the uterus (a partial hysterectomy).

You really have three treatment choices with fibroids because they have such a clear relationship with excess oestrogens, or excess sensitivity to oestrogens. The first course of action that your doctor may offer you is a intra-uterine coil which uses synthetic progestogens to try to control the impact that oestrogens are having on the fibroids. The second choice is the one already discussed, which is surgery with all its attendant physical, and possibly mental, traumas. The final option is to consider using natural progesterone in tune with your cycle, as suggested by Dr John Lee, the leading expert on the use of natural progesterone, and the author of *Natural Progesterone: A Remarkable Hormone*. This has the effect of opposing oestrogen and reducing its impact on sensitive tissues. In this way the fibroids can be decreased in size and kept at a low and non-disruptive level until the menopause. When you go through the menopause they will naturally shrivel up.

ENDOMETRIOSIS

With endometriosis, small fragments of the lining of the womb – endometrial tissue – work their way through the muscular wall of the womb, through the fallopian tubes, and then attach themselves to other organs and the body cavities around them. They can be found everywhere from the ovaries to the bowels. These tissue fragments respond to cyclical hormonal events in the same way as if they were still lining the uterus. This means that premenstrually they fill with blood and then, during the period, they bleed into the cavities around them. This can cause considerable pain, and the discomfort can continue for several days. Lesions can also form on all the surrounding areas, including the fallopian tubes and the bowels. It is common, too, to experience pain at ovulation time and sometimes during sexual intercourse, plus going to the bathroom can be uncomfortable, not necessarily just at the time leading up to menstruation. Endometriosis is often the cause of infertility, especially if pregnancy is delayed to beyond the age of 30, and around 40 per cent of women who report infertility turn out to have some endometriosis.

One in ten women suffer from endometriosis during their reproductive years, and it typically takes seven years to diagnose. Frequently, young women are put on the Pill to contain heavy or painful periods, and yet taking the Pill has been shown to double the likelihood of developing endometriosis. The causes of this painful disease are unknown. There has been an increase in its incidence, and some experts refer to it as exclusively a 20th-century disease, suggesting that the lifestyle or dietary changes that have occurred in the last few decades, and/or the introduction of chemicals into the environment, have had a strong influence. The American Endometriosis Association has made links between environmental pollutants, called dioxins, and the sharp increase in this disease. Some women find that pregnancy resolves the problem, or at least makes huge improvements in it. It also may be worth wearing looser trousers and underwear as tight clothing has also been implicated in endometriosis. The belief is that the corset-like pressure leads to reflux of the endometrial tissue up through the fallopian tubes into the abdominal cavity. Again, the menopause normally signals the end of endometriosis, though damage from lesions can leave some residual problems in severe cases.

Conventional treatment of endometriosis may centre on prescribing synthetic progestogens, to emulate the condition of pregnancy. The other usual treatments are surgical, and laser surgery usually retards the progress of the disease for a short while, but does not cure it. Hysterectomy may resolve it, but can be a traumatic solution for a young woman. Treatment with natural progesterone, which is a molecule that is identical to progesterone manufactured in the body, may be more appropriate in terms of not unsettling the body's fine balance. Dr John Lee has had a good deal of success treating endometriosis with natural progesterone and he recommends that it is used from day six through to day 26 of the cycle, using a total of 25 grams of cream per week for the three weeks. Dr Lee claims that this measure stops the symptoms worsening and causes the pain to subside over a period of six months, but admits that it contains rather than cures the problem.

As with other inflammatory diseases, saturated fats from meat and dairy products and hydrogenated fats from margarines and packaged foods can increase inflammation, and animal fats are also a significant source of exposure to dioxins. Fish oils and nut, seed and vegetable oils help to reduce inflammation. This is important for endometriosis because inflammation occurs at the sites where the endometrial tissue attaches to other structures and this is probably why the discomfort is felt. It may take a few months for the pain to subside and the monthly bleeding to lessen, and so allow the sites which are inflamed to heal. Alongside this it is strongly advised that you reduce exposure to all sources of environmental oestrogens by following the advice in **Cut Out Chemicals**, page 61. The object of these steps is to reduce inflammation and the effect of oestrogens. It is also important to support the immune system, and you can read about measures which help immune function in **Thrush and Cystitis** on page 112 and **Pelvic Inflammatory Disease** on page 145.

Other nutrients which have been shown to help with this condition are vitamin C, which helps to reduce inflammation, and B-vitamins, which assist with bringing down the inflammation and also help the liver to break down oestrogens. Take three grams daily of vitamin C with bioflavanoids, preferably in the form of magnesium ascorbate, calcium ascorbate or potassium ascorbate, and 100 mg of a B-complex daily. The healthy fats described in Point 1 of the 7-Point Plan are particularly anti-inflammatory in their action and you may want to take extra supplements to help to bring the condition under control.

OVARIAN CYSTS

Cysts in the ovary can grow to the size of a chicken's egg and, while they are sometimes symptom free, can also result in considerable pain. One in five women investigated have ovarian cysts.

Ovarian cysts are the result of an egg failing to develop normally, but continuing to grow. It continues to be sensitive to the effects of luteinising hormone (LH), which influences the site of the cyst to swell. This can result in pain, and even in bleeding at the site. Infertility drugs have been implicated in a proportion of cases. These drugs encourage an increase in follicle stimulating hormone (FSH) and LH, which can aggravate the condition. Conventional treatment usually centres on surgery and not all surgeons will remove the egg without removing the ovary.

A lack of zinc may result in a woman being more susceptible to ovarian cysts because zinc is needed for the normal development of eggs. Natural progesterone can also be used to treat ovarian cysts, and it is taken from day 10 through to day 26 of the cycle. This has the effect of stopping ovulation, which gives the ovaries a rest and the time to heal. This is often sufficient to shrink the cysts successfully over two or three cycles, after which no further treatment is needed.

POLYCYSTIC OVARIES

Polycystic ovary syndrome (PCOS) involves too many male hormones – androgens – being produced, and this blocks the normal development of egg follicles. As a result, the ovaries become enlarged and covered in unruptured small cysts containing undeveloped eggs. The increased male hormone levels mean that PCOS can be linked to male pattern hair growth, including that on the face. Other symptoms can include irregular periods, male type weight gain (i.e. apple shape instead of pear shape), and an enlarged clitoris. It often affects other hormone levels with high luteinising hormone (LH), low progesterone and either high or low oestrogen. Around 20 per cent of women are affected, but most mildly. About 7 per cent develop more serious symptoms, including weight gain, irregular periods, excess hair, acne and conception difficulties. Measuring hormone levels with a blood test can be helpful, but it is most useful to have an ultrasound to identify if PCOS is the problem. It is not uncommon to be prescribed the Pill, or anti-androgenic drugs, to alleviate some of these symptoms, or for fertility treatment to be suggested if the woman would like to conceive. The herb, saw palmetto, which is usually used successfully to treat prostate enlargement in men, also has a significant use for the treatment of PCOS. This is because saw palmetto interrupts the conversion of testosterone into DHT (dihydrotestosterone) which is the troublesome form of the male hormone. Saw palmetto seems to positively affect the symptoms of PCOS such as male pattern hair growth. Take 300mg twice daily.

There is a strong relationship between PCOS and a blood sugar problem called insulin resistance. This means that the advice given about blood sugar regulation in **Balancing Blood Sugar Levels** on page 104 is very relevant to women with PCOS. Low progesterone relates to high LH levels and high testosterone levels, and this explains why natural progesterone is a very useful treatment option for PCOS.

PELVIC INFLAMMATORY DISEASE (PID)

PID is the general term given to serious inflammation of the uterus and the fallopian tubes. Abscesses can result which lead to considerable pain. PID is also a cause of infertility. The development of the disease usually starts in the vagina and cervix, and then the infection creeps further up the reproductive tract. Bacterial infections, such as chlamydia, which is responsible for two-thirds of PID cases, are normally treated with antibiotics. If PID is severe, surgery may be suggested. Lowered oestrogen levels, as a woman nears the menopause, can reduce the mucus in the vagina, and this can make her more susceptible to infections. PID can cause scarring (adhesions) which cause the pelvic organs to stick together and not function properly. It can cause blocked fallopian tubes and increase the risk of ectopic pregnancies. As one in four women have PID at some point, this makes it very important to have it diagnosed early.

Boosting the immune system to help the body to resist opportunistic organisms which lead to infection is the first priority. Following the 7-Point Plan is an excellent foundation, and there are immune-enhancing foods which can help considerably. These include dark red, blue and purple berries, garlic, onion, live yoghurt, the spice turmeric, seaweed (which can be milled and used as a salt substitute) and ginger. Ensuring you eat these foods at every opportunity can make quite a difference. There are also certain nutrients and supplements which help to keep the immune system boosted. The most useful of these are vitamin C, along with the other antioxidant vitamins A and E, the minerals zinc and selenium, quercitin and some herbals: echinacea, cat's claw tea, aloe vera and astragalus. Drinking at least

2 litres of water daily is also important to support the immune system. Reduce, or even better cut out, stimulants and sugar as these profoundly affect the immune system.

CERVICAL EROSION AND DYSPLASIA

Cervical erosion is when the cells lining the cervix are affected and replaced by a different type of cell (squamous epithelium are replaced by columnar epithelium). Contributing factors can include infection or trauma, such as childbirth. Early treatment is advised (by cauterisation, cryo surgery or douches) to reduce the risk of it leading to cervical cancer.

Cervical dysplasia is more commonly termed pre-cancerous. When this is diagnosed a close eye is kept on it, but it is not always treated as it may not progress to full-blown cervical cancer. If it is, cauterisation is the most common treatment. Smoking, hormone imbalance and vitamin deficiency have all been linked to cervical dysplasia. Routine cervical screening has improved the opportunity to catch early stages of cervical cancers, however screening is imperfect and will miss around five per cent of cases. A form of cervical cancer which is increasing among younger women is adeno cancer. This develops in the glands of the cervix rather than on the surface, making it harder to detect. The fact that screening can be faulty makes it even more important to take preventive measures against this disease.

High doses of folic acid – 10 mg for at least three months, against the normally suggested intake of 200–400 mcg – have been shown to improve dramatically, or totally reverse, cervical dysplasia. It is always best to take a B-complex alongside large doses of any one B-vitamin (which folic acid is). Vitamin A and beta-carotene levels in women who develop cervical dysplasia tend to be lower than average, and other vitamins and minerals are also known to help: vitamin C, B6, selenium and magnesium. Using a programme of 3–5 mg of folic acid, along with 50 mg of B6 and 300 mg of magnesium has been shown to help reverse the condition. You can also use some natural progesterone cream and/or oestriol cream internally between periods. Artificial progestogens do not have the same effect because they dry up the cervical secretions, which may lead to an acceleration of the problem.

Self-treatment for cervical dysplasia, such as I have just described, must not take the place of medical advice, but is worth considering if your doctor has advised a wait and watch approach.

STAYING AWAY FROM THE SURGEON'S KNIFE

Medical intervention can be pretty drastic with women undergoing hysterectomies for complaints such as heavy bleeding and fibroids. This 'spare part' surgery views the female reproductive organs as being troublesome, with no particular further use, and considers it acceptable to 'whip them out'.

Many women endure hysterectomies simply because they are unaware of any other option. The number of these operations is increasing each year, with one in five women in the UK currently having a hysterectomy by the age of 65. Two-thirds of the 90,000 annual operations are carried out because of heavy periods in younger women, and not as a life-saving procedure. This is quite a heavy price to pay on such a grand scale and, of course, for the individual woman the operation can be traumatic. There are strong socio-economic trends attached to the likelihood of having a hysterectomy, with women who leave school without qualifications being 15 times more likely to have the operation compared to women with a degree. This suggests that sufficient information is not being given or getting through to these women.

Over the past few years a new technique, microwave endometrial ablation (MEA), has emerged with the aim of finding a procedure which will help to reduce the rate of unnecessary hysterectomies performed on women with heavy periods. In this procedure the lining of the womb is cauterised to reduce the amount of bleeding. A recent trial has confirmed the superiority of MEA over other surgical procedures.

If it is proposed that you have a hysterectomy to deal with heavy periods, fibroids or endometriosis, you always have the option of treating it using the methods described above for several months first. If your health is in crisis to the point where surgery is being contemplated, it is essential to follow the dietary advice rigorously to achieve best results. It is not much use, say, to only partly give up caffeine. To ward off surgery you will have to give it your best shot. And if you do decide to go for surgery these measures will also have the effect of preparing your body for surgery so that you go into the operation in the best possible condition for an early recovery.

Another, less drastic, procedure that is performed on many women is the D&C – dilation and curettage. This has been carried out since 1843 and, while it is portrayed as being a routine operation, it must be remembered that any procedure that requires a general anaesthetic is not minor. A D&C can be carried out both for investigative purposes and for therapeutic reasons. It may be used therapeutically, for instance, to remove uterine growths or after a miscarriage. However, when it is used for investigation, or for blind biopsies, it is worth realising that in 75 per cent of cases D&Cs do not show up anything at all, probably because the majority of problems turn out to be hormonal. You can usually avoid an investigative D&C if you ensure you are referred to a specialist trained in ultrasound imaging, a painless and accurate procedure using a vaginal probe with fluid-enhanced sonohysterograph.

CANCERS OF THE REPRODUCTIVE TRACT

These cancers – cervical, ovarian and endometrial – are all hormone related, as are the majority of breast cancers. Even men do not escape lightly, with testicular and prostate cancers having a hormonal connection which is likely to be linked to oestrogens. Men can also have hormone-related breast cancer. I have already discussed in **Oestrogen Overload** how the impact of our natural, but over-strong, oestrogens, along with exposure to environmental oestrogens can have an impact on hormone health.

This new wisdom linking hormones to certain cancers was not available only a few decades ago. Oestrogen-only HRT was first linked to a 20-fold increase in the risk of developing endometrial cancer. Endometrial cancer tends to occur in the five to ten years before the menopause. During this time anovulatory cycles are more common – these are cycles when an egg is not produced, and therefore no progesterone is produced. Eating sources of phytoestrogens during this ten-year phase, along with a generally healthy diet, should do a lot to reduce the risk of endometrial cancer according to many experts.

Ovarian cancer is also on the increase and affects around two per cent of women. It is closely allied to the same set of conditions which have been linked to breast cancer, and they even share the same genetic risk factors, with the same genes being a factor in ten per cent of cases of both ovarian cancer and breast cancer.

We now have widespread screening programmes, which means that conditions such as cervical cancer can be picked up at an earlier stage than previously. There are many influencing factors on these conditions, and the links between diet and cancers have shown than increased fruit and vegetable intake is beneficial for prevention, and that high saturated fat intakes have a strong negative association.

Because hormone-related female cancers are strongly allied to high oestrogens, or unopposed oestrogen levels, it should help to achieve hormonal balance, by decreasing damaging excess oestrogens. Here is a checklist of factors you can influence:

- Decrease excess exposure to environmental oestrogens
- Increase dietary levels of phytoestrogens
- Reduce levels of fat in the diet, especially hydrogenated and saturated fats
- Raise levels of fibre in the diet
- Include exercise in your programme
- Lower alcohol intake
- Breastfeed for at least three months, and preferably a year, as it reduces the risk of ovarian and breast cancers.

CHAPTER TWENTY

Managing Your Menopause

The menopause is called 'The Change' for a reason. It is a time when fundamental physiological shifts happen to a woman, often accompanied by changes in other aspects of her life – perhaps the children have grown up and left home, retirement may beckon, maturity inevitably brings a different perspective on life and maybe more energy is needed for the onslaught of boisterous grandchildren. Since one-third to one-half of a woman's life will be lived after her menopause these days – she might as well enjoy it!

Handling the physical symptoms and health issues associated with the menopause is one positive step that you can take to ensure that you enjoy this time, and the years that follow it, to the full. Various health matters come to the forefront which all relate to changing hormone levels. The most important are the increased risks of osteoporosis and an increased risk of heart disease. Of more immediate concern, during the time of hormonal fluctuations, are symptoms such as hot flushes, decreased libido and vaginal dryness. All of these have a foundation in hormonal shifts.

At the menopause the levels of oestrogen drop to around 40 per cent of the levels that are produced during a woman's reproductive life, while progesterone drops to only about one per cent.

There are many ways that dietary manipulation can improve menopausal symptoms and risk factors. In the East, in countries such as Japan, China and Singapore, there are considerably fewer menopausal-related problems compared to the West. Factors in their diet predispose them to a 'change' which is barely noticeable. There is not even a word for hot flushes in the Japanese language.

IS SOYA NATURAL HRT?

Soya is, as we have already discussed, a source of phytoestrogen isoflavones. These can help to balance the oestrogens we produce in our bodies, and can probably also help to counter the effects of environmental oestrogens. In addition, they have a hormone replacement effect once our own natural oestrogen supplies begin to wane. The mild oestrogen effect of soya can ease menopausal symptoms for many women, without creating oestrogen-related problems. The oestrogenic effect of soya isoflavones is probably what accounts for the scarcity of menopausal symptoms in countries such as Japan, where large amounts of soya are eaten.

Various studies support this theme and have shown specific effects from intakes of soya phytoestrogens. One study showed that 50 grams of soya protein daily led to a 33 per cent reduction in the number of hot flushes after only four weeks, and a 45 per cent reduction after 12 weeks. In another study, menopausal women with an average of 14 hot flushes per week each, supplemented their diets with wheat or soya flour each day and experienced a reduction in hot flushes by 40 per cent over three months. These are extremely positive results to achieve in such a short time. If plant oestrogens, which we can get from soya, wholegrains and legumes are incorporated into the diet in a significant way for a longer time during the peri-menopause phase then even better results may be expected.

COOLING HOT FLUSHES

Hot flushes can be very troublesome for some women, who can experience them up to ten or even 14 times in a 24-hour period. Night sweats can cause you to wake up in the night drenched with sweat and with soaked sheets. The time taken to towel down and change linen can be a major interruption to sleep leaving you feeling exhausted the next day. Sometimes the pulse can race up to 150 beats per minute.

Caffeine, alcohol and high stress levels are all implicated in worsening hot flushes. Hot flushes are rare in vegetarian societies, suggesting that vegetables and legumes are protective and that meat consumption may aggravate the situation. Hot flushes may be due in part to low levels of endorphins in the brain – our pleasure chemicals. Levels of endorphins can be improved by exercise. Stress management also helps to rectify endorphin levels.

It can be helpful to take a supplement of 800 ius of vitamin E for at least three months to see if this improves the situation. It is effective for about 50 per cent of women but if, after three months, the vitamin E is not helping, it is necessary to try other tactics. Vitamin E should not, however, be used at this level if you are taking blood-thinning medication such as Warfarin, as it can thin the blood further. Other supplements can help: 2 grams daily of vitamin C with bioflavanoids in the formula. It is best to take a non-acidic version such as magnesium ascorbate or potassium ascorbate. Magnesium (300 mg daily) and folic acid (400 mcg daily) have also been found to provide relief, as have evening primrose oil, starflower oil or borage oil giving 200 mg of GLA. Several herbal preparations can help, and these are listed in **Herbs for Harmony** on page 85.

Practical advice also encompasses using divided, layered bedding, so that you can throw off covers while your partner remains covered up. Cotton bedding is far more comfortable than any other option. Keep your surroundings cool and well ventilated, as hot rooms and central heating can trigger hot flushes. It is also an idea to keep a spray bottle of water near you, to use on your face and wrists.

EXERCISE

Regular exercise is important at all stages of life, but it has particularly important health ramifications for women approaching, and beyond, their menopause. Weight-bearing exercise is one of the more important factors in reducing the risk of osteoporosis, while the links between a healthy cardiovascular system and exercise have also been established without question. Exercise has positive effects on blood pressure, blood fats, cholesterol and blood sugar control – all of which affect cardiovascular health.

It has also been shown that women who are sedentary are more likely to have moderate or severe hot flushes when compared to women who exercise.

You are never too old to start an exercise programme, and after only ten weeks of regular sessions a moderate degree of fitness can be achieved. If you are particularly unfit, or have existing severe osteoporosis it is best to consult your doctor before beginning a programme.

MENOPAUSAL WEIGHT GAIN

Women who are post-menopausal are inclined to put on a few extra kilograms, but this is usually true weight gain rather than bloating. It is normally the case that older women are less active, meaning that they put on weight more easily. Their hormone balance also alters to favour a change in the ratio of male to female hormones, which encourages fat deposition around their middles instead of around their hips.

Hormone replacement therapy (HRT) will frequently encourage bloating simply because of the continued exposure to oestrogens. At a time when oestrogen levels are meant to be dropping, they are boosted again artificially by HRT.

A HEALTHY HEART

One of the concerns which post-menopausal women need to contend with is that their risk of cardiovascular disease becomes similar to that for men. The number of strokes (blood clots or haemorrhage to the brain) in women post-menopausally are worse than for men and, in 1995, accounted for 13 per cent of female deaths against eight per cent of male deaths. The protective effects of their hormones ceases to have an influence. For this reason HRT is often suggested to menopausal women as a way of reducing their risk of strokes and heart attacks. But heart disease, as with other diseases, does not just creep up on you the day you stop menstruating. There are many predisposing factors which lead up to the moment you experience the heart attack or stroke. These are mainly: smoking, lack of exercise, stress and diet. So, at best, hormone levels are protective, but not necessarily causative factors. And in any event, most women do not manage to stay on HRT for more than a year – while any protective benefit is only felt after seven years of use.

Risk Factors for Cardiovascular Disease

Advancing age	Family history of heart disease	Stress
High blood pressure	Low physical activity	Diabetes
Overweight by 20 per cent	Abnormal cholesterol levels	Smoking
More than 3 units of alcohol daily	Menopause, especially early or surgically induced	High salt diet
		Low fibre diet

All the measures mentioned so far in this book will help to reduce the risk of heart disease. It is particularly important to address fibre levels in the diet, and to eat the helpful fats. Oily fish and fresh nuts have been shown to have a significant impact on heart disease risk. A diet high in fruit and vegetables, at least five portions daily, is one of the most protective measures, with people in countries with high consumption of these foods having the lowest rate of cardiovascular problems. Not smoking is vital, and exercising sufficiently to get slightly 'puffed-out' four times a week is highly protective.

There is another strong risk factor for heart disease which is of great interest to post-menopausal women. It is estimated that one in four men and post-menopausal women have a genetic predisposition to a condition called homocysteineuria. This means that an essential amino acid, methionine, is broken down into a compound called homocysteine at a greater rate than normal and this is then not adequately processed by the liver. Homocysteine is a toxic compound which has been strongly implicated in cardiovascular disease and Alzheimer's. It may also be linked to osteoporosis. It is likely that a woman's hormones before the menopause protect her to a large degree against this condition, but she loses the protection post-menopausally.

Some of the B-vitamins are effective at getting the process of detoxifying homocysteine going again. These are folic acid, B12 and B6. A 50–100 mg strength B-complex may be one of the cheapest ways of preventing these crippling diseases in a large number of the population, including post-menopausal women.

It is wise not to take iron supplements post-menopausally unless you know yourself to be anaemic. It is thought that one of the factors which protects pre-menopausal women against heart disease is that they menstruate and so lose iron in the blood. Free-iron can cause oxidation damage and affect the arteries. Men who give blood, and so lose iron, seem to share this protective factor with menstruating women.

REMEDIES FOR OTHER COMMON MENOPAUSAL PROBLEMS

Headaches and migraines often become worse with the menopause. Avoid trigger foods which contain amines: cheese, wine, oranges, chocolate, yeast, pickles, alcohol. Other triggers are commonly eaten foods such as wheat, diary products and caffeine.

Insomnia can be a problem, especially if hot flushes and night sweats are keeping you awake. Obviously, dealing with the hot flushes is the first step, but the herb valerian can help to induce sleep, although it should not be taken alongside other sedatives.

If mild to moderate depression is a problem at this time, it is well worth using the herb St John's wort, but not alongside other antidepressants. Taking kava kava helps to curb anxiety.

Dry vagina problems can impact upon libido. Natural progesterone often helps, but if it is more persistent using some oestriol (E3) cream internally can help. Phytoestrogen-rich foods such as soya have been shown to have a beneficial effect on vaginal tissue. An active sex life also helps to keep vaginal tissues healthy by improving blood flow to the area. If sex becomes uncomfortable, use a lubricating gel. Drinking lots of water, 2 litres daily, helps to keep tissues hydrated.

Memory loss is often reported and, once again, addressing blood sugar problems may be the best remedy. B-vitamins are important for memory function, and the herb gingko biloba helps to combat problems with an effective memory.

PROGESTERONE AND THE MENOPAUSE

Oestrogen and progesterone levels plummet at the menopause. While there seems to be a consensus amongst the medical profession that it is helpful to replace oestrogens, progesterone has been largely forgotten about. This is possibly because it is so strongly identified with child-bearing, which obviously ceases to be relevant.

During our evolution we did not live long enough, on average, to get beyond the menopause, and so it could be considered that we did not have a need of these hormones – but we now live well beyond our forties and fifties, meaning that for optimal health we may need to review this position – but not necessarily with artificial hormones. The second issue is that we are now surrounded by a sea of oestrogens from pharmaceutical, agricultural, petrochemical and other environmental sources, such as plastics. These xenoestrogens, which are likely to be affecting our hormone health, need some opposition. This is where progesterone may come in.

Natural progesterone used in the peri-menopausal and post-menopausal phases has been shown to increase bone density and improve cardiovascular health. The cream has also been used to reduce hot flushes, improve libido and combat vaginal dryness. It may be the case that, if natural progesterone is not successful on its own, some oestriol cream may need to be used alongside it. Oestriol is the type of oestrogen which is not involved in an increase in risk of hormonal cancers. See **Natural Hormones** on page 91.

CHAPTER TWENTY-ONE

Reversing Osteoporosis

One in three women over the age of 60 will break a bone due to osteoporosis, and up to one-third of bone mass can be lost. HRT is often suggested as a preventative measure for post-menopausal women to avoid this disease. And yet at best HRT only delays the problem and merely protects them while they are taking the drug and shortly afterwards. They then lose the benefit and research has shown that at age 75–80 women who have taken HRT have almost the same risk of breaking a bone as women who never took the drug.

Bone consists of living tissue and is permanently undergoing a cycle of renewal. This means that the opportunity to maintain bone health is good if you address the health aspects which are known to support bone regeneration.

There are many different factors associated with bone health, and hormone levels are one of the most important. Low levels of the hormones oestrogen and progesterone accelerate the loss of bone tissue post-menopausally, and it is the low levels of oestrogen that HRT seeks to address.

Osteoporosis is sometimes called the silent thief, because it sneaks up unannounced stealing bone tissue, until one day, usually later in life, a hip or wrist is broken, or vertebrae crushed. This can lead to a degeneration in health to the point were many people die directly as a result of such a breakage. The scary thing about this is that it is all going on invisibly inside, and most people do not have the faintest idea if osteoporosis is a likely problem for them. It is not only women who have osteoporosis. While one in three women develop osteoporosis, around one in eight men develop it.

The disease is the result of loss of mineral density in bone tissue. Bones become thinner with age in most people, but in some this process is accelerated and more severe. There are three main types of fractures that happen with osteoporosis. The first is apparent in a loss of height and results in the stoop or hunch that is seen in a lot of elderly women. This is caused by vertebral crush, where the vertebrae collapse under the minimal stress of lifting an object, or even simply under the stress of the body's own weight. The second type commonly occurs when breaking a fall with the hand and the bones of the wrist or forearm fracture. The final type is the most serious and this is the hip fracture. Up to half of elderly people end up being nursed full time after breaking their hip, and a fifth of people with hip fractures will die within a year from complications.

It is easy to have a bone scan and it can be the best way of either putting your mind at rest, or of finding out if you need to do something about the problem. A bone scan uses such low-dose radiation that the technician stays in the room, and while it is not cheap, it is certainly less expensive than the problems associated with breaking bones. Your doctor can arrange for you to have a bone scan if you ask for one, though he/she may be unwilling to do it on their own budget. Alternatively you can have a simple urine test which assesses bone turnover. It can tell you about current levels of bone loss and assess the risk of future loss. It is excellent for monitoring the effects of diet and supplementation on bone turnover but does not tell you the actual condition of your bones.

RISK FACTORS FOR OSTEOPOROSIS

Osteoporosis is a complicated issue and addressing the problem by assisting hormone levels is one major way of seeking to avoid it. There is an increased risk of osteoporosis with hormonal events such as an early menopause or a history of many missed periods. However, there are many other factors which are involved in increasing the risk of osteoporosis. Here are the main ones:

- The risk of osteoporosis increases with age.
- People who are shorter and have small frames are more likely to develop osteoporosis than people who are taller and heavier.
- Smoking leaches calcium out of the bones.
- Alcohol leaches calcium out of the bones.
- A high daily intake of salt leaches calcium out of the bones.
- Calcium and magnesium balance in the diet are important and we will look at this in more detail later.
- Vitamin D helps calcium to be taken up by the bones more effectively. We now know that vitamin K is also important and we will look at these two vitamins in more detail later.
- Too much phosphorous, found, for example, in carbonated soft drinks, upsets calcium/magnesium balance, and leaches calcium out of the bones.
- Weight-bearing exercise, such as skipping, using a trampoline or fast walking taxes the bones sufficiently for them to be triggered into building themselves up against the regular assault and is one of the most important protective factors against osteoporosis. Non-weight-bearing exercise, such as cycling or swimming, does not have this effect. Take your doctor's advice if you already have osteoporotic fractures.
- Chronic stress causes calcium to be released from the bones and dumped into the hair.

- Excess protein from the diet causes calcium to be leached out of the bone. This has serious implications for those who drink large quantities of milk and we will discuss this later.
- Excessive use of the hormone thyroxine beyond the body's need for it reduces mineral levels in bone. If you are prescribed thyroxine by your doctor, it is essential to have the levels checked regularly to avoid an excess of thyroxine.
- A history of anorexia or bulimia can lead to osteoporosis. Women in their thirties can suffer fractures of the spine or other bones if they have had a history of severe eating disorders.
- Long-term use of steroid medication.
- Previous fracture from a slight injury.

BONE BUILDING

Cells called osteoclasts are responsible for carrying away old bone tissue – like dumper trucks carrying away old building materials from a building site. Cells called osteoblasts have the job of renewing bone by depositing minerals in the holes which have been left behind by the osteoclasts – like cranes filling in the gaps with cement blocks that fit the building design.

Bone density peaks at around the age of 35 in women and then begins to decline slowly. After the menopause the decline in bone density accelerates for around ten years. Later this bone loss continues but at a slower rate.

Many hormonal factors influence the body's ability to build or to break down bone tissue, and oestrogens and progesterone balance is just one of them. The hormones which directly affect the osteoclasts and osteoblasts are actually produced by the thyroid and parathyroid glands. These hormones are called calcitonin and parathormone. The health of the thyroid gland is therefore important when considering hormone and bone health.

Interestingly, oestrogens, which are routinely prescribed for bone health, do not regenerate bone at all. Their actual function is to stop mineral loss from the bones, and while this helps, it is not the whole answer. The female hormone which is responsible for encouraging mineral absorption into the bones is progesterone.

DOES DRINKING MILK HELP OSTEOPOROSIS?

Calcium is the main mineral in our bones and it is widely recognised that 1000 mgs daily is the amount that post-menopausal women need to have in order to help maintain bone density. This means the average woman, who gets around 500–700 mg daily from her diet, will need to supplement 300–500 mg.

Women are advised to eat or drink a lot of dairy products, in order to achieve a higher dietary intake of this key mineral. We are also told to take vitamin D to improve absorption of the calcium. As we have already found, osteoporosis involves many factors and this advice is too limited to yield really promising results. Indeed, we in the UK have continued to see an increase in osteoporosis despite having one of the highest consumptions of dairy products in the world. The missing link is magnesium. Milk is rich in calcium, but has very low levels of magnesium. The body is unable to use calcium fully unless it is in the correct balance with magnesium.

Since around 10–15 per cent of white people and 60–90 per cent of people from other ethnic backgrounds can be allergic to milk or have lactose intolerance, the advice to drink milk may often be contrary to best health. In many cultures where dairy products are not a significant part of the diet, and calcium is low by Western standards, osteoporosis rates are nevertheless lower than for people in developed countries such as the UK, US and Australia.

It is interesting to reflect that cows grow to meet their large genetic potential, not by drinking their own milk, but by eating grass. And here we have a clue. Green leafy vegetables give the ideal balance of minerals for bone health, including calcium, magnesium and boron. Nuts and seeds are also superb storehouses of these minerals.

A major 12-year study of nearly 8000 women, reported in the US in 1997, concluded that women who drank two or more glasses of milk daily had a significantly greater risk of hip and forearm fractures than did women who drank one glass of milk or less per week.

Controlled trials have shown that when magnesium was included with calcium there were overall increases in bone density beyond those which would be expected with calcium alone. If you take calcium supplements it is best to take magnesium alongside them. The most useful ratio is double the quantity of magnesium to calcium for six months to a year, to rectify any magnesium deficiency, followed by equal amounts of magnesium to calcium thereafter. This would translate into 600 mg magnesium to 300 mg calcium, followed by 500 mg magnesium and 500 mg calcium. It is best to use calcium citrate and magnesium citrate rather than other types of minerals. Calcium carbonate, for instance, is simply chalk.

If you want to continue to include dairy produce in your diet make sure you choose low-fat varieties. It is of greater value to eat live yoghurt than to drink milk. Many milk-intolerant people can tolerate yoghurt as much of the lactose has been predigested. Yoghurt is also a good source of B vitamins, produced by the bacteria, the minerals are more easily absorbed, and it is a useful source of beneficial bacteria which help bowel health (this in turn can promote vitamin K production – see page 166).

Non-dairy sources of calcium (per 100 gms/ml)

Sprats	700 mg	Broccoli	100 mg
Sea vegetables (i.e. kelp)	400–1200 mg	Haddock	100 mg
Canned sardines	400 mg	Beans and pulses	70–100 mg
Enriched flour	200 mg	Oranges	80 mg
Almonds	200 mg	Dates and raisins	75 mg
Figs	200 mg	Carrots	50 mg
Canned salmon	150 mg	Wholewheat bread	50 mg
Tofu (calcium enriched)	150 mg	Eggs	50 mg
Enriched soya milk	140 mg	Apples	35 mg
Green leafy vegetables	100–170 mg	Blackberries	35 mg

VITAMIN D

The 'sunshine vitamin' is so called because we are able to manufacture it in our skin when we are exposed to sunlight. It is vital for depositing calcium in our bones and if we do not get sufficient sunlight exposure we need to make sure either that we eat a diet rich in vitamin D, or that we take supplements – 400 ius daily if you are often out of doors, 800 ius if you are not. Sunlight exposure, leading to vitamin D synthesis, has also been shown to positively influence the incidence of breast cancer dramatically. Food sources of vitamin D are sardines, herrings, salmon, tuna, egg yolks, fish oils, dairy produce. Interestingly, studies have not shown that dietary vitamin D helps, but this is probably due to the fact that most of the dietary vitamin D comes from dairy produce, and you can see my comments in the section above about dairy produce. It is likely that fish sources of vitamin D are more beneficial.

BEEFING UP YOUR BONES?

Protein is a vital constituent of our diet, but in a typical Western diet we do tend to overdo it. The Government agencies recommend that we have around 44 grams daily of pure protein, but on average we eat more like 80 grams. The problem with this from the point of view of osteoporosis is that protein makes the body acidic. Minerals are then needed to restore alkalinity in the cells. Calcium is used for all the steps in this process and the primary way the body sources this mineral is to leach it from the bones. If we are eating an excess of protein, this means that more calcium is being robbed from our bones than we are able to replace. This is one of the main problems of the advice to drink milk for calcium. Milk is also a major source of protein, which means that while we get some calcium benefit, it is also being taken out of the bones to deal with the protein.

VITAMIN K

Until recently, this was mainly thought of as the vitamin that helps blood clotting and its other benefits were largely ignored. Now, however, Vitamin K is being seen in a new light as it is apparent that it is critical for bone health. We manufacture vitamin K in the bowels and it has always been assumed that because of this it is not necessary to supplement it. So many people on a Western diet have impaired bowel health that it is likely that a large number of them have lowered vitamin K manufacture. Vitamin K is essential for a substance called osteocalcin, which is the protein matrix upon which mineralisation takes place in the bones. It provides correct structure and order to bone tissue and so vitamin K plays a key role in the formation, repair and remodelling of bone. Without strength, this calcium structure becomes fragile and, like chalk, breaks easily. Prothrombin tests which pick up vitamin K deficiency may not be subtle enough to detect mild vitamin K deficiency which may be sufficient to damage bones. Food sources of vitamin K include: cauliflower (the best source), yoghurt, alfalfa, egg yolks, safflower oil, kelp, fish liver oils, leafy green vegetables, potatoes, milk. Supplements are available, though not widely, and one 100 mcg tablet daily should be more than sufficient.

LOW STOMACH ACIDITY

Stomach acid (HCl) is necessary to liberate minerals from food, and from supplements, and this includes all the bone-building minerals – calcium, magnesium, phosphorous, boron and zinc – as well as iron, manganese and other minerals. If we have insufficient levels, this can be a major contributing factor to a poor mineral profile. While people are commonly diagnosed with high stomach acidity, low acidity is barely recognised, and yet a high proportion of people who visit nutritionists have this problem. It is made worse with advancing years, with an estimated 60 per cent of people over the age of 50 having low stomach acidity. Gastric tests have shown that those with osteoporosis can have 50 per cent of the stomach acidity of people without osteoporosis. Signs of low HCl levels can include weak and brittle nails, a heaviness after eating protein meals, constipation and indigestion, but often there are no symptoms at all. You can buy HCl (with pepsin) supplements and take them with your meals. Take one, and build up to five supplements with a meal. Do not take them if you have ulcers or reflux (a tendency to acidy burps), and discontinue taking them if you get a burning sensation. You can neutralise any such sensation immediately by drinking milk. However, this reaction is rare, and it is more often the case that HCl supplements help a wide range of digestive problems, as well as mineral uptake. You can take digestive enzymes alongside them for general digestive health. After a while your stomach should have improved its own production and you can step down the number of supplements you take, though the older you are, the more likely it is that you will need to take some in perpetuity.

OTHER FACTORS

Once again a diet high in fruit and vegetables is probably one of the important protective factors. They are high in vitamin C, which is involved in building the bone matrix, as well as collagen and cartilage. An additional two grams daily of supplemented vitamin C may also be helpful.

Soya foods have been shown, in trials, to improve bone density post-menopausally. This evidence is in line with other information that soya has a mild oestrogenic effect.

The mineral chromium has been shown in studies to reduce the loss of calcium in the urine by 50 per cent in post-menopausal women, while at the same time improving their oestrogen levels. Taking 200–500 mcg daily may help osteoporosis, and will also help to balance out blood sugar levels.

Onions have been shown in recent research to be even more beneficial than other foods in increasing bone density in rats. The rats were fed dried onion every day for a month and, compared to those fed soya, milk, other vegetables and herbs, they developed much stronger and thicker bones.

THE LEE STUDY

As already mentioned, Dr John R Lee of California, US, is the person who has published the most information about natural progesterone. He conducted an interesting study with 100 women aged 38–83 (average age 65.2). Most of the women had already suffered spontaneous vertebral fractures leading to height loss. Where appropriate the women were prescribed oestrogens, but a third of the women could not be prescribed oestrogen as they had medical conditions such as a history of breast cancer, high cholesterol or clotting disorders. All of the women received three per cent progesterone cream to use for the second half of their cycles (or to mimic this if post-menopausal). They continued for three years. All of them were given other advice: to increase consumption of green leafy vegetables, to reduce intake of alcohol and red meat, cut back on smoking, and exercise three times a week. They were also advised to take vitamin and mineral supplements, including calcium and vitamins D and C.

In all the women height loss was stabilised and no further osteoporotic fractures occured. In 63 of the 100 women their bone density was checked every 3–6 months (the other 37 women found the cost of the tests prohibitive). Normal expectations would have been for an average of 4.5 per cent bone loss over the three years. However, every one of the 63 women tested had an increase in bone density, many substantially more than would have been expected by other means. In the group as a whole, average bone density improved by 15.4 per cent, with the same results observed in 70-year-old women as in younger women. The women receiving oestrogen and progesterone did no better than the women receiving progesterone only. It is possible that progesterone alone is effective because it can be converted to oestrogen if needed.

Three women broke bones due to falls while hiking, in a car accident and falling downstairs. All healed particularly well, despite two of the three women being in their seventies and eighties. Critics of natural progesterone grudgingly concede that this study is interesting, but do comment that the dietary advice may have been instrumental in the results, and that no control group of women taking a placebo was used. Yes, diet may have been a factor, and this should be a message to all that no one measure works alone.

Several independent studies to evaluate Dr Lee's work are now under way, but results are not yet available. Only one placebo-controlled trial has published results so far, and it found that there was a significant improvement in hot flushes associated with the menopause (83 per cent of women using the cream versus 19 per cent using a placebo cream). However, the trial found that there was not much difference in bone density after one year (19 per cent of women using the cream versus 17 per cent of those using the placebo – both groups were also given dietary and other advice). However this trial used only 1/4 teaspoon of natural progesterone once a day, and it is likely that slightly higher doses administered twice daily is ultimately found to be a more useful level (see the dosage suggestions in **Natural Hormones** on page 91). Obviously more controlled studies are needed.

CHAPTER TWENTY-TWO

Closing Thoughts

Women's reproductive health is so important to their families. They are the ones who will house a growing life for nine months, and their partners suffer alongside them if they have premenstrual problems or menopausal discomfort. The national budget can suffer as well. If a woman has to be medicated in the long term, if she develops osteoporosis with all the implications for care in later years, if cardiovascular health is a problem, or breast cancer is diagnosed, again these cost the Government a fortune – as well as the woman much distress, even perhaps her life, and her family a lot of heartache.

Prevention is undoubtedly better than cure, and thankfully women are beginning to take the matter into their own hands. Well-Woman clinics have started the process of self-awareness, but often these clinics serve only to reinforce the message that artificial hormones are the solution to the symptoms, and do not really focus on discovering the root causes.

So much good can be done by addressing dietary and lifestyle factors that it is a shame that this is often not the first course of action undertaken, but the last. Enjoy your good health, and your transition to balanced hormones. If you benefit, do tell other women, because it is still the case that the majority prefer to keep intimate problems to themselves, yet it is only by spreading the word that other women will find out what is possible.

Part Six

APPENDICES

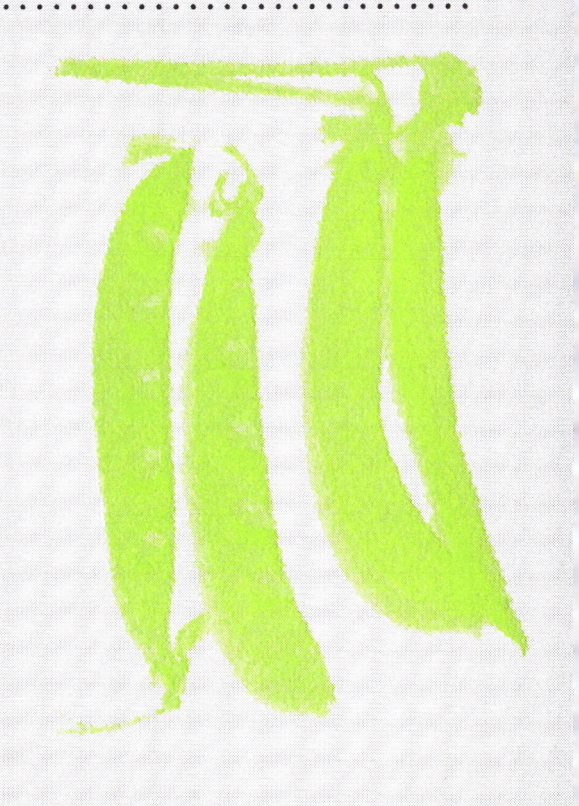

Note the days you menstruate by highlighting or marking with M, or use the chart for menopausal symptoms. Note any symptoms you experience with a code you decide upon. For instance: B = breast tenderness, H = headaches I = irritability, C = cramps, HF = hot flushes, HB = heavy bleeding, SC = sugar cravings, W = water retention. You could also give it a score. For instance: 1 = mild, 2 = moderate, 3 = severe.

You can use this chart to better understand the patterns of your symptoms and to monitor how they improve. Feel free to copy these pages as you need to.

MONTHLY CHART — Year:

	Jan	Feb	Mar	Apr	May	Jun
1						
2						
3						
4						
5						
6						
7						
8						
9						
10						
11						
12						
13						
14						
15						
16						
17						
18						
19						
20						
21						
22						
23						
24						
25						
26						
27						
28						
29						
30						
31						

Appendix I

MONTHLY CHART — Year:

	Jul	Aug	Sep	Oct	Nov	Dec
1						
2						
3						
4						
5						
6						
7						
8						
9						
10						
11						
12						
13						
14						
15						
16						
17						
18						
19						
20						
21						
22						
23						
24						
25						
26						
27						
28						
29						
30						
31						

Appendix II

SOURCES OF FIBRE

Listed below are common sources of fibre from fresh foods. To find the fibre content of packaged foods, look on the nutrition panel which will give the amount per 100 grams or 100 ml serving. Check to see how much your serving portion actually is.

Foods which have no, or trace amounts of, fibre

Meat, poultry, fish, eggs, dairy products, fats and oils, confectionery, most beverages (vegetable or fruit juices, and soya, rice or oat milks, may have some fibre)

Foods which give around 0.5 grams of fibre

- 100g   tofu
- 50g   asparagus, melon, pineapple, tomato
- 25g   French beans, cabbage, carrots, cauliflower, celery, cherries, fresh figs, lettuce, strawberries

Foods which give around 1.0 grams of fibre

- 2   average apricots
- 1   medium peach, medium plum
- 100g   cooked white rice
- 50g   cooked barley, rhubarb
- 25g   white bread, broccoli, Brussels sprouts
- 15g   blackberries, currants, chestnuts, raisins, sunflower seeds, walnuts

Foods which give around 1.5 grams of fibre

- 100g cooked brown rice
- 50g swede
- 25g raw beetroot, uncooked oatmeal, peas, cooked spinach
- 15g blackcurrants, dried dates, peanuts
- 10g almonds

Foods which give around 2.0 grams of fibre

- 1 tbsp linseeds
- ½ medium avocado pear
- 1 medium apple, medium banana, medium orange, medium pear
- 100g white cooked spaghetti, whole potatoes
- 50g cooked lentils, parsnips, yam
- 25g wholemeal bread, plantain, raspberries
- 15g fresh coconut

Foods which give around 3.0 grams of fibre

- 100g white flour
- 50g cooked butter beans, cooked haricot beans, cooked buckwheat (kasha), cooked chickpeas
- 15g dried figs, dried prunes

Foods which give around 5.0 grams of fibre

- 1 medium corn on the cob
- 100g rye flour

Foods which give around 10.0 grams of fibre

- 100g wholemeal flour
- 100g soya flour
- 100g cooked wholemeal spaghetti

Resources

To find out more about Suzannah Olivier's activities see her website at:
www.healthandnutrition.co.uk
EMAIL: eattobefit@aol.com

HERBAL AND NUTRIENT SUPPLEMENT SUPPLIES

SOLGAR Herts 01442 890355
- Stocked by good independent health food shops.
- Nutrients: a large range of low to high dose vitamins, minerals, essential fats and digestive aids.
- Female health: Omnium, Prenatal Nutrients, genestein (from soya), iproflavone, Isoflavone Concentrate, Herbal Female Complex. Also supply a range of herbal supplements. Those for female hormone balance include alfalfa, dong quai, agnus castus (chasteberry), black cohosh.

BIOCARE Birmingham 0121 433 3727
- Stocked by good independent health food shops. Direct mail ordering service also available.
- Nutrients: large range of vitamins, minerals, essential fats and digestive aids.
  Mixed ascorbates is a good powdered buffered vitamin C with flavanoids.
- Female health: Soflavone, Femforte I and II, Phytosterol Complex.
- Bone health formula: Osteoplex.

HEALTH PLUS East Sussex 01323 737374
- Direct mail ordering service available.
- Nutrients: range of quality nutrients. Also supply convenient Daily Packs. Each contains a combination of supplements that are designed for specific health conditions. There are 28 daily packs in each box.
- Female health: Menopause Pack, Pregnancy Pack.
- Bone health formula: Joint Pack.

HIGHER NATURE East Sussex 01435 882880
- Direct mail ordering service available
- Nutrients: range of vitamins, minerals, essential fats and digestive aids. As well as flax seed oil and Essential Balance Oil, which are an excellent alternative to other salad oils, they also supply coconut butter.
- Female health: nenophase, Mexican yam, Soyagen.
- Bone health formula: Osteofood.

LAMBERTS Kent 01892 552120
Available from good independent health food retailers
- Nutrients: large range of vitamin, minerals, essential fats and digestive aids.
- Female health: Genovite Plus, alfalfa extract.
- Bone health formula: Osteoguard.

NUTRI High Peak 0800 212742
- Nutrients: large range of vitamin, minerals, essential fats and digestive aids.
- Female health: Menobalance, Prenatal phase 1, 2 and 3.
- Bone health formula: Osteo-P-Complex

THE NUTRI CENTRE London W1 020 7436 5122
- Stock a wide range of nutrition products, health foods and books from various suppliers and manufacturers. They also have their own range, NutriWest. You can visit the shop and all their stock is available by mail order.

TO FIND A NUTRITIONAL THERAPIST

BRITISH ASSOCIATION OF NUTRITIONAL THERAPISTS
Tel: 0870 6061284
BCM BANT London WC1N 3XX
For a list of registered nutrition therapists please send a large S.A.E. to BANT at the above address.
INSTITUTE FOR OPTIMUM NUTRITION Tel: 020 8877 9993
I.O.N., Blades Court, Deodar Road, London SW15 2NU
For a directory of nutritionists, send £2 to the above address.
SOCIETY FOR THE PROMOTION OF NUTRITIONAL THERAPY Tel: 01582 792088 P.O. Box 85, St Albans, Herts AL3 7ZQ
For information please send SAE and £1 to the above address.

WOMEN'S NUTRITION ADVISORY SERVICE Tel: 01273 487366
www.wnas@wnas.org.uk
Information, advice and self-help books on all aspects of women's hormonal health, including dealing with menopausal symptoms without HRT or coming off HRT safely. The WNAS offers 'scientifically based tailor-made programmes'. Clinics in London and East Sussex. Postal and telephone consultations available.

SUPPORT GROUPS

THE NATIONAL OSTEOPOROSIS SOCIETY (N.O.S.)
Tel: 01761 471771 www.nos.org.uk P.O. Box 10, Radstock, Bath BA3 3YB
N.O.S. offer support to people with osteoporosis, their families and carers through a range of information booklets, a helpline and a network of over 100 regional support groups.

SHE (SIMPLY HOLISTIC ENDOMETRIOSIS) Tel: 01522 519 992
www.shetrust.org.uk Red Hall Lodge, Red Hall Drive, Bracebridge Heath, Lincs LN4 2JT

NATIONAL ENDOMETRIOSIS SOCIETY Tel: 0207 222 2776
www.endo.org.uk 50 Westminster Palace Gardens, Artillery Row, London SW1P 1RL

ENDOMETRIOSIS ASSOCIATION INTERNATIONAL HQ (USA) www.endometriosisassn.org/default.htm

NATURAL FAMILY PLANNING AND PRECONCEPTION

FERTILITY EDUCATION TRUST Tel: 01222 754 628
218 Heathwood Road, Cardiff CF14 4BS

NATURAL FAMILY PLANNING TEACHERS ASSN
Tel: 07931 651 326 Linked to Fertility Education Trust, above.

NFP CENTRE Tel: 020 7371 1341 Clitheroe House, 1 Blythe Mews, Blythe Road, London W14 0NW

FORESIGHT For information and a list of Foresight practitioners, write to: The Old Vicarage, Church Lane, Witley, Godalming, Surrey GU8 5PN

BOOKS

Natural Progesterone Dr John R. Lee, John Carter Publishing, 1999
Natural Progesterone AnnA Rushton & Dr Shirley Bond, Thorsons, 1999
The Breast Cancer Prevention and Recovery Diet Suzannah Olivier, Michael Joseph, 1999

Endometriosis – The Key to Healing Through Nutrition Dian Mills, Element, 1999

Our Stolen Future T. Colburn, D. Dumanoski, J. Peterson Myers, Abacus, 1996

The Feminization of Nature Deborah Cadbury, Hamish Hamilton Ltd, 1997

What Doctors May Not Tell You About The Menopause Dr John R. Lee, Warner Books, 1996

Preventing and Reversing Osteoporosis Dr Alan R. Gaby, Prima Books (California, USA), 1994

The Case for Preconceptual Care for Men and Women Arthur and Margaret Wynne, ABC Academic Publishers, 1991

RECIPE BOOKS

Cooking Without Barbara Cousins, HarperCollins, 1997
Oestrogen The Natural Way – Recipes for the Menopause Nina Shandler, Villard, 1997
The Optimum Nutrition Cookbook Patrick Holford and Judy Ridgeway, Piatkus, 1999

NATURAL PROGESTERONE INFORMATION AND SUPPLIES

THE WELL WOMAN'S INTERNATIONAL NETWORK
Tel: 07000 437225 (touch phone service for information and membership)

NATURAL PROGESTERONE INFORMATION SERVICE (NPIS)
NPIS, P.O. Box 24, Buxton, Derbyshire SK17 9FB
Send S.A.E. for a list of doctors who are familiar with the use of natural progesterone.

HIGHER NATURE Tel: 01435 882880
Supplies natural progesterone to medical doctors. Pro-Gest Cream and Pro-Gest oil.

BIOCHEMICAL TESTING

Most of these tests are only available through practitioners. It is strongly advised that for those which are available direct to the public, that they are interpreted by a nutritionist or other health professional so that results of the test can be acted upon appropriately.

APPENDICES

AERÓN LIFECYCLE LABORATORIES (USA) Tel: 001 510 7290375
Saliva tests for female hormone levels.
Aeron hormone saliva tests are also available through Higher Nature (01345 882880)

DIAGNOSTECH LTD Swansea 0800 731 5655
Female hormone profile (saliva).

GREAT SMOKIES DIAGNOSTIC LABORATORY
The services of this laboratory can be organised through their UK agents, Diagnostic Services Ltd, Tel: 0151 922 6200. Female health profile (saliva) and osteoporosis profile (urine).

THE INDIVIDUAL WELLBEING DIAGNOSTIC LABORATORY London SW3 Tel: 020 7730 7010
Osteoporosis profile (urine).

ORGANIC FOOD SOURCES

THE SOIL ASSOCIATION Tel: 0117 929 0661 Bristol House, 40-56 Victoria Street, Bristol BS1 6BY
The Soil Association can provide a list of organic suppliers in the UK, as well as publications on organic issues. Telephone for a copy of their free catalogue.

DISTILLED WATER SUPPLIERS

WHOLISTIC RESEARCH COMPANY Tel: 01707 262686
www.holisticresearch.com
HIGHER NATURE Tel: 01435 882880
AQUAPURE DISTILLATION Tel: 020 8892 9010
FRESHWATER FILTER COMPANY Tel: 020 8597 3223
THE FRESHWATER COMPANY Tel: 0345 023998
www.freshwateruk.com
Delivery service of pre-distilled water in the south east of England.

CHEMICAL-FREE COSMETICS AND HOUSEHOLD PRODUCTS

THE GREEN PEOPLE Sussex 01444 401444
A range of natural cosmetic products. Mail order and also available from health food shops.

THE NATURAL COLLECTION Tel: 01225 44 22 88
www.greenstore.co.uk P.O. Box 2111, Bath BA1 2ZQ